CONSCIOUS BIRTHING

*Yoga and Meditation
for Pregnancy*

CONSCIOUS BIRTHING

Yoga and Meditation for Pregnancy

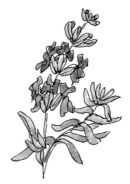

Theresa Jamieson

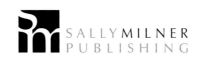

SALLYMILNER
PUBLISHING

Sally Milner Publishing Pty Ltd
734 Woodville Road
Binda NSW 2583 AUSTRALIA

© Theresa Jamieson 2009

Design: Anna Warren, Warren Ventures Pty Ltd
Editing: Anne Savage
Photography: Creative Jungle
Illustrations: Beth Nelson
Index: Deirdre Ward

Printed in China

National Library of Australia Cataloguing-in-Publication entry

Author:	Jamieson, Theresa.
Title:	Conscious birthing : yoga and meditation for pregnancy / Theresa Jamieson.
ISBN:	9781863513913 (pbk.)
Series:	Milner health series
Notes:	Includes index.
Subjects:	Hatha yoga
	Meditation
	Exercise for pregnant women.
Dewey Number:	613.7046

Disclaimer
Information and instructions given in this book are presented in good faith, but no warranty is given nor results guaranteed, nor is freedom from any patent to be inferred. As we have no control over physical conditions surrounding application of information herein contained in this book, the author and publisher disclaim any liability for untoward results.

10 9 8 7 6 5 4 3 2 1

CONTENTS

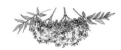

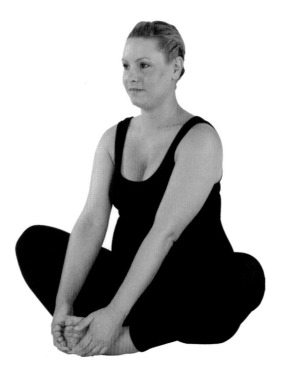

FOREWORD

As a young and inexperienced doctor, I first trained in a large city obstetric hospital. Even then, I was amazed at the high level of 'problem pregnancies' and intervention in labour.

When I left the city to work in the country, it became obvious that the management of pregnancy and labour was much different, with intervention less necessary. It was a lesson in how different the process of pregnancy and labour can be when the woman was relaxed and surrounded by 'at ease' staff and supportive family and friends.

After thirty years of being in general practice, I've found that the whole concept of preparation and labour has changed. It includes many more disciplines of care, and other skills and resources.

Yoga is one of the new disciplines that can enhance skills for the preparation of childbirth. It also encourages the development of skills that will be useful in parenting, and for immediate as well as subsequent personal, physical, emotional and spiritual aspects of life.

It has been obvious to me that women practising yoga for the childbirth preparation carry a new, and different dimension into this role, and their lives in general.

Theresa's book reflects this changed approach, and celebrates her own life and broad experience. Her extensive practice and teaching of yoga, in particular with regard to pregnancy, childbirth and parenthood is apparent.

She expresses this experience readily to her readers, while her passion for the subject and her universal knowledge in what she writes about, produces a uniquely helpful reference and training manual for any woman about to prepare for pregnancy.

All women, and their support teams, would do well to read and practise the guidance illustrated in this lifetime work.

Dr Robert Tiller
MB, ChB, DipObs, DCommH

ACKNOWLEDGEMENTS

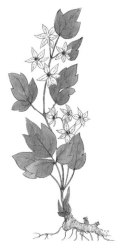

Firstly I would like to thank my publisher, Libby Renney, for giving me the unexpected opportunity to to write a second book including the concepts of conscious birthing and the importance of living each brief moment as it happens, especially the moments of transient nature that are pregnancy and the life of a baby in its mother's womb. It had always been my dream to bring new life to my book and to once again share with pregnant women the extraordinary value that yoga and meditation has during this precious time, and to share what pregnant women have taught me about pregnancy yoga since I began teaching in 1984. It has been a constant joy to bring this information to birthing women in the hope that they will be encouraged to embrace their pregnancies and have a positive attitude about birthing. Without Libby's support and positivity my dream might never have become a reality. I also want to thank the editor, Anne Savage and the designer, Anna Warren, who gave my book an easy to understand format while maintaining the physical and spiritual nature of pregnancy and birth. Many thanks to Brian Usher and Daniel from Creative Jungle for their excellent photography. A special thanks to Bec and Elizabeth who gave their time to do the photos so late in their pregnancies and to Madyanti who did the post natal photos so beautifully just 5 months after Sita was born. I am also very grateful to the women who contributed inspiring birth stories and lovely photos.

A special thanks to my beautiful sons Ezra and Reuben, just because they are my beautiful sons. Without them I would never have discovered the wonderful joy that is pregnancy and the true blessing that I have in being their mother. Without them I would never have experienced that aspect of being a woman or the unlimited value that yoga has to offer during pregnancy, childbirth and as a life skill. Heartfelt thanks to my mother, who has always been a constant support, and as she is my mother I feel it appropriate to dedicate my book to her. Thanks go to my brother Peter, who is always encouraging and who, I think, is quite chuffed to have his wife Sue and his sister as published authors. My sincere thanks to my dear friends, especially Robbie, Erma Linda, Sandra, Suzanne, Debbie and Cheryl, and to Eileen for her help with getting some structure into my writing time. Thanks also to Paul for his constant support and sincere enthusiasm, and to Chris and John, who have always been so positive about my endeavours. And a special thank you to Quazz, who introduced me to yoga. All these people were more helpful than they were aware and have all helped to keep my spirits and confidence up when moments of self-doubt inevitably flooded my consciousness.

This book is really the result of the confidence shown to me by my doctor in Auckland, John Barrett, who was present at the birth of Ezra and whose suggestion it was to organise a pregnancy yoga class for me. His fulfilment of that promise and continued support while I was living in Auckland were to be the beginning of my specialising in this gentle form of yoga. I am ever grateful to him for his belief in me and what had so helped me during my pregnancy and birth experience, and for his genuine faith in my work with pregnant women. A very special thank you to the many, many women I have had the privilege to teach since that time, who have definitely taught me more about what aspects of yoga really are the most suitable for pregnant women—I could never have known this from my own experiences. They have been, and continue to be, a constant source of information and inspiration of the unlimited benefits that are available through yoga. Being with them during these special days of pregnancy provides a constant reminder of the true wonder of being a woman with child and the miracle of a new life within them. Many thanks also to the doctors and other medical professionals on the Gold Coast who have continued to support my works with pregnant women and birth preparation since I began teaching here in 1987.

My understanding of yoga would be far less if I had not had the good fortune to meet my wonderful teachers Shantimurti and beautiful Bhaktinmurti, who were always inspirational and totally believed in the many benefits that were available through the practice of yoga. Their extraordinary knowledge, understanding and instruction are my foundation in yoga and meditation and the traditional practices detailed in my book. And finally to my beautiful dogs Kunga, Stella Nova and Mos for their unconditional love and patience as I needfully neglected them to dedicate my time to writing—especially to Mos, who became instantly depressed when he saw me turn on the computer, knowing that meant no long walks or games to be played for many hours thereafter.

Dedication

For my wonderful mother Josephine Mary: love to you always.
All mothers carry within their womb the blessing and wonder of a precious new life.
My book is in their honour: they nourish and bring forth the miracle of life.
And in loving memory of my father, my husband Jeff and beautiful Annastasia.

INTRODUCTION

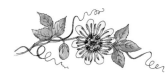

Birth: A Celebration of Life

Pregnancy is a brief and remarkable time in your life as a woman—both transient and immensely transformational, a time in which you evolve from one aspect of being a woman to another, of being a mother. From the moment of your child's conception you will be in your new role of caring for this life within you and, just as your baby changes constantly in your womb, so too will you in your body and your mind, and in every aspect of your life. This is a unique and precious time, one where you have the opportunity to really honour and nourish yourself as a woman on every level of your being— mind, body and spirit. It is also the beginning of a new relationship, one that begins the moment your womb provides the safe environment for the newly fertilised ovum from which your baby will evolve.

It is disappointing that so many first-time mothers are completely put off the idea of natural childbirth, often because they are ill informed and overloaded with birth stories that were in some way difficult. It is a reality that some women won't even consider the possibility of a natural birth—it just isn't an option for them, taking the pain relief available as soon labour begins. There is no judgement in that, only a little sadness that there is not enough encouragement and education about how empowering birth can be. Birth is painful, but I have heard many women say it was easier than expected. I wonder if women were left to their inherent natural ability, and were willing to trust more, they might be in awe of what birth is rather than having no confidence in this natural process. Maybe if we didn't have any preconceived ideas about birth, it might be viewed in a very different light.

The media doesn't help alleviate women's concerns either. Many movies which include 'birth scenes' portray the woman on her back, in pain and terribly distressed. These scenes become imprinted in our psyche and can be hard to shift. But consider the movie *The Blue Lagoon*, in which two children grow up unaffected by such images. They are innocent and naive to the fact that sex is connected to conception and that when a woman is pregnant her body changes dramatically— naturally and beautifully. Because they had no prior knowledge, the young girl went into labour naturally and gave birth with that innocence, lacking fear and self-doubt. Although it's Hollywood, some women have found this movie quite helpful, as it encourages them to look at birth in a different, more positive way.

One of the most beautiful ways to look after yourself and your unborn baby is through gentle yoga practices and meditation outlined in this book, selected with your needs as a pregnant woman foremost in mind. The different yoga techniques—the postures, the breathing and meditations—provide you with an opportunity to truly care for yourself to be there with your baby in your womb. This is a wonderfully calm way to nurture yourself during your pregnancy and in preparation for a completely new life when your child is born.

I want to emphasise that this book is for the benefit and enjoyment of *all* women who are pregnant, whether the birth of your baby is a straightforward vaginal delivery or whether it eventuates that you need medical intervention, or whether for personal or medical reasons your labour results in a caesarean delivery. Birth is birth. However your baby moves from the environment of your womb into our world, it is the bringing forth of a totally new life. You have carried and cared for your baby since you first realised you had conceived, and although the birth is of great importance, it is not the only essential to have your attention on. Both natural birth and caesarean birth are awe-inspiring, resulting in the blessing of a new life and one of life's most incredible moments, and both can be gentle, calm and incredibly beautiful, the birth of a completely new soul with its own unique personality and personal destiny. After birth, life naturally goes on and you will be in your role of mother for the rest of your life, always caring and wondering about the welfare of your son or daughter. The skills explained here and the benefits they so generously give are there for every part of your pregnancy and for every women and her own set of circumstances and birth experience. The practices outlined have been successfully used during the birthing process for both vaginal and caesarean deliveries. Many of the women I teach have natural unassisted births, some in their homes and others in hospital, some in water and others on land, while others give birth through caesarean. No one way makes you a better mother or guarantees that your baby will grow into a better person, for there are many other factors that influence the journey to life in the outside world.

This book comes partly from my own experiences during pregnancy, but primarily from the privileged time I have had teaching yoga and meditation and the concept of conscious birthing to pregnant women since 1984. It reflects my intense desire to share the many worthwhile benefits that yoga and meditation offer to all women during pregnancy and in preparation for birth, and to share knowledge of the practices which will prove invaluable after the birth as life skills. This is one of the most nourishing ways to care for yourself during your pregnancy—for your mind, your body and your soul—and for the baby in your womb. The rewards are there no matter how fit you are or if you are completely new to yoga.

Women are individuals, and I cannot guarantee that practising yoga during pregnancy will be the wonderful experience for you that it has been for most of the women I have met. However, if a little time is given to understanding and learning the different techniques I recommend, I am confident it will make a favourable contribution to your pregnancy, to the birth of your baby and to your recovery. Practising yoga while you are pregnant will give you the space to come back to yourself, to discover a very peaceful and gentle awareness at the very centre of your being and to be there with the precious new life in your womb. When yoga is done with complete breath and body awareness and a clear and conscious mind state, is like coming home to yourself.

The specific yoga practices that will benefit you during your pregnancy and preparation for childbirth include the yoga postures or *asanas*, the most valuable breathing techniques or *pranayama*, the importance of breathing consciously, and meditation, including traditional practices and some lovely creative visualisations.

The exercises and postures have been chosen because they are specific for you at this time and take into consideration your ever-changing needs and requirements. They are very gentle and always safe and are explained with the necessary modifications included to accommodate the changes that occur. They will strengthen and tone your body as your progress through your pregnancy and help you to maintain flexibility and a sense of wellbeing, and also help you to recover more easily after the birth. A number of these exercises are excellent in helping to overcome some of the more common problems that accompany pregnancy, while others are excellent to use during labour. It is not necessary to have practised yoga before this to enjoy the many wonderful benefits they have to offer. The pelvic floor exercises that are

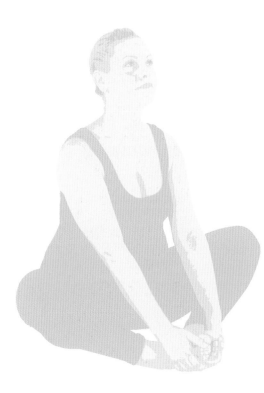

an important aspect of all pre- and post-pregnancy care are also discussed in detail.

Yoga breathing practices are in many ways the most important aspect of your birth preparation. They bring about metal calmness and physical relaxation, which enable you to better cope with the demands of childbirth. The simple yoga breathing exercises embraced during pregnancy have been used by many women as a primary coping strategy during labour; they are empowering and encourage more confidence and strength from within.

Meditation and relaxation together form an invaluable part of yoga. Both evolve naturally from the yoga breathing exercises and are a main component of birthing consciously. They are very closely linked but different—without being able to relax, meditation is not possible. Meditation and inner reflection provide you with the opportunity to embrace your pregnancy, to be mindful of the wonder of the life growing inside your womb and to realise how special it is to spend time alone and at peace with yourself and with your baby. Relaxation and meditation allow you the space to simply be—to be still, to feel calm, steady and strong. Through these gentle practices you will develop confidence and courage from within yourself and, importantly, become more conscious of the present moment.

In Part IV, Complementary therapies, I discuss the use of aromatherapy during pregnancy and birth and its value

when used with some gentle massage techniques. These techniques are an excellent way for your birth support to care for you during pregnancy and labour and a lovely way for them to be more involved in the birthing process. Some provide relief from minor back problems and help to overcome pain, others are very gentle and more relaxing in nature. Water birth is a very gentle approach to childbirth. I have included information on it and an inspiring water birth experience as more and more women are choosing to labour and give birth in this way. I also briefly explain the principles of hypnobirthing and how it can be used as a birth skill, especially with the help of your birth support. I have studied hypnosis and hypnobirthing and discuss the similarity in procedure and results to yoga. I feel the benefits are increased greatly when it is used in conjunction with the yoga breathing techniques and other mindfulness practices.

Part V, Conscious birthing, begins with a chapter on the role of your birth support, outlining how your birth support can best assist you. Chapter 19, Skills for birth, is intended to help you use the breathing practices and some of the relevant yoga postures during labour. I briefly discuss the role of hormones during labour and birth and how your ability to stay calm and relaxed influences their fine balance. I explain the importance of three key words—*trust, surrender* and *accept*—and how reflection on them has often made a shift to a more positive mind state so useful to a birthing woman and her birth support.

Some very inspiring and interesting birth stories come from women who have used many of the practices detailed in this book to their benefit during their birth journeys. It is very encouraging for newly pregnant women to read what other women used during their birthing experiences, what gave them the most relief from pain and the skills that gave them courage and confidence.

In Part VI, At home with your baby, I outline comprehensive yoga programs for the first six months after birth. This is a gentle and very enjoyable way to slowly incorporate yoga into your life again using a natural progression of exercises. Many are from the antenatal section but because you are no longer pregnant I have excluded the modifications for pregnancy and included some other relevant postures. This becomes a complete yoga program valuable for women of all ages. I explain the importance of continuing with relaxation, the breathing exercises and meditations wherever possible to help alleviate stress and fatigue and to encourage mental and physical health. I hope this will inspire you to continue to take care of yourself and be nourished through yoga long after the birth and as you move forward into the joys and challenges of being a mother.

Conscious Birthing

The concept of conscious birthing has proven to be the strength behind women managing childbirth in a positive and fulfilling way, whether a natural home birth or a hospital delivery with intervention. In essence it is a combination of the traditional yoga breathing practices and a clear understanding of meditation, together with being mindful of yourself, your pregnancy and of your baby in your womb.

Conscious birthing is in part using two powerful forces during childbirth—the ability to stay clear and focused, and an understanding of the ancient yogic teaching of the breath. This combination encourages women to approach birth with more confidence and courage, to surrender to the enormous energy of birth and the wisdom to trust in themselves more fully, and ultimately to birth consciously and intuitively.

Conscious birthing is also about reflecting on the life of your baby in your womb and embracing the miracle that

is happening to you as a woman, and a mother. It is about being mindful of the transformation that is taking place within you, in your body, your mind and your soul, moment to moment. This very gentle approach to pregnancy and childbirth allows you to get in touch with your inherent feminine wisdom and the energy of birthing women and mothers throughout time, and to embrace this brief and remarkable time in your life.

The concept of conscious birthing is relevant in every pregnancy and for every birth. All the practices detailed here are invaluable for pregnancy, the unknowns of labour and as skills for the rest of your life. It is my hope that you will enjoy and benefit from these gentle concepts in all aspects of your life, so that you have a conscious pregnancy, a conscious birth experience and include these skills into living your life consciously as well.

When the mind is used in conjunction with the breath it gives a woman the tools she most needs to move through the birthing process with a centred mind and positive attitude. This gives her the confidence and courage to surrender to whatever occurs during childbirth, to trust in herself and her birth support, personal and medical, and to accept whatever unique circumstances the birth brings. Trust. Surrender. Accept.

Conscious birthing is empowering—it strengthens the mind, and draws you home to yourself and to your baby in your womb. It also brings to light that this time in your life is not only a very physical journey but also a very spiritual one. The purpose is to encourage the best way for you to stay well and healthy during pregnancy in every aspect of your self and to move through the birthing process as gently, calmly and confidently as possible—and ultimately to embrace being a mother with the same awareness and positivity.

While the information here is based on the ancient traditional yoga teachings and practices, it also includes feedback from the many women I have taught. Pregnant women are very intuitive and know better than anyone what feels right and what they gain the most benefits from. It is

their opinions about the teachings that are the life of this book, simply because they learnt them, they became skilled with them and then used them with confidence and often extraordinary courage to birth their babies. I have always trusted their opinions and listened to what was most beneficial for them. They have taught me more about yoga for pregnancy than I could have imagined, helped me to refine the practices and respectfully modify the wonderful traditional teachings to a system that pregnant women respond to and benefit from the most. Having seen the positive results I am eager to share my own experiences as a teacher and what has helped countless women during pregnancy and childbirth, and given them something to trust in as they move through their new lives as mothers.

Women are pregnant for approximately 37 to 42 weeks and the birth can last from as little as one or two hours, sometimes less, to more than a day. When the time comes for a woman to give birth she wants to feel confident that she and her baby are safe and supported. She also wants to know how best to cope, how to breathe efficiently and how to remain as relaxed and together as possible, and this is best done by knowing how to relax, how to breathe and how to breathe consciously.

I believe, like many, that your child has chosen you as its mother and that beyond birth you have a journey together until the end of your days. Being a mother will last your whole lifetime. Although the

techniques are primarily for pregnancy and birth, most mothers would agree that carrying a baby and giving birth are the easy part. These simple techniques will benefit you during the comparatively brief days of pregnancy and birth, and hopefully become skills to use for a lifetime.

It is my hope that whatever the circumstances of your birth journey you feel strengthened and encouraged, that you are proud of yourself as a new mother, with a fresh found confidence, and that you remember to be aware moment to moment and to embrace your life with joy and wonder. Conscious birthing is empowering and nourishing to you in every aspect of yourself, your mind, your body and your spirit that brings these extraordinary brief moments more fully to your awareness.

Thoughts on Caesarean Birth

The way your baby comes into this world from the world inside your womb is a unique and incredible moment. It is natural to want it to be as peaceful and calm as possible—but birth is definitely in the realm of the unpredictable. In truth, with all the yoga and breathing in the world it can sometimes be very different to how you might have wished. For this reason I want to talk about birth through caesarean, which for many women is an unwelcome and devastating outcome after months of thinking they would birth differently. I feel it is important to see it as a possibility, so that if it does occur the grief of not having a natural birth experience will be less and hopefully easier to come to terms with. Many times women are just not prepared for this unexpected outcome and often haven't even considered it, but not to do so can lead to enormous distress and disappointment.

It is important to remind yourself that however the birth occurs you have given life to a new soul who you will continue to care for in every way simply because you are the mother and always will be. The need for an emergency caesarean can arise even when labour seems to progressing well and a natural birth is seemingly inevitable, but through no fault of anyone the procedure is required—either to save your baby's life, or yours. When this occurs it is obviously very stressful for the birthing woman and understandably very disappointing.

Some other women for very personal reasons might elect for a caesarean birth, either fully conscious or under general anaesthetic, but this in no way diminishes her love for her baby or her ability to care and nourish her child in the days before and following the birth.

The view of many is that caesarean deliveries are often done when it really isn't necessary. There are doubtless some situations where if a woman had been encouraged to move through the labour differently and had felt more confident within herself, she could have delivered her baby vaginally. There is also the reality that many women just don't feel they can give birth naturally, so fearful of the pain they won't even contemplate giving normal labour a chance. It is interesting that many women who have given birth naturally are surprised it was in reality less painful than they had anticipated.

A few weeks before she was due, a student in one of my classes brought her sister along with her, a theatre nurse who had been present at many caesarean births. When caesareans came up as a topic of conversation after the class she felt qualified to comment. In the past when we had discussed caesarean birth it was often viewed with a hint of negativity. If a woman knew she was to deliver that way for medical reasons she often felt very disappointed and was not as supported as she could have been. When a woman chooses a caesarean for personal reasons it sometimes elicits judgements from family and friends, an unfortunate situation but very much a reality. There is a very real pressure, often from other women, to birth naturally and sometimes it just doesn't happen that way—the emphasis is too often on the method of delivery rather than on what this is really all about—a new baby, a precious new life. Our visitor's thoughts on this subject were insightful and a very positive way to look at a fairly common occurrence. She said that although not a natural birth, a caesarean birth was still beautiful, it was birth, the awe-inspiring moment that a new soul, a child comes into the world and takes its first breath. In her mind birth was always remarkable, a sacred moment in life, and she always felt honoured to be present. Since that time I have often told this story as a way to remind my classes that a caesarean is as much a birth as a vaginal delivery, it is an exquisite and beautiful experience in life. You have given birth to your baby.

No matter how well prepared a woman is, very little will ease the disappointment if a natural birth doesn't eventuate. A more positive, less rigid attitude can help change the energy around this outcome and if you believe in destiny, that is just how it was meant to be, then disappointment can be replaced with acceptance and most importantly the joy of a new life.

Throughout the book I talk of 'being present', of realising the preciousness of life and living life in the moment—of being mindful of the brief time that is pregnancy and to hold in your mind how quickly your baby is changing in your womb, and even more apparently once she is born. To be aware of the transient nature of all things can encourage us to live our lives with awareness in every moment, to be awake to life more often, and to do so with gratitude and appreciation for the blessings that life brings, even among the lesser moments. And because pregnancy and infancy are particularly brief they are the perfect opportunity to be as one with each moment, as often as possible.

It has always been a great joy for me to meet young mothers and see them nourished through the gentle practice of yoga and meditation during this brief and unique time in their lives, encouraging them to be conscious in their pregnancies and to birth, and live that way too. This work came to me not through conscious choice, but was really given to me and is a gift in the truest sense. It has been a constant blessing and has taught me so much more about the wonderful benefits that yoga and meditation have to offer to everyone, as well as giving me an opportunity to appreciate the transient nature of my own life, my children's lives and those dear to me, and of life itself.

A beautiful quote from renowned author Deepak Chopra holds the essence of what I am attempting to say here, and as always he does it so eloquently. His words not only emphasise the transient nature of all life but capture what conscious living and birthing is about. This heartfelt excerpt from *The Seven Spiritual Laws of Success* illustrates the very 'spirit' of being present, of living life well, and living with gratitude and love:

We are travellers on a cosmic journey— stardust, swirling and dancing in the eddies and whirlpools of infinity.
Life is eternal. But the expressions of life are ephemeral, momentary, transient.
Gautama Buddha, the founder of Buddhism, once said.
'This existence of ours is as transient as autumn clouds,
To watch the birth and death of beings is like looking at the movements of a dance.
A lifetime is like a flash of lightening in the sky,
Rushing by like a torrent down a steep mountain.'
We have stopped for a moment to encounter each other, to meet, to love, to share.
This is a precious moment, but it is transient. It is a little parenthesis in eternity.
If we share with caring, lightheartedness, and love, we will create abundance and joy for each other. And then this moment will have been worthwhile (page 111).

And finally a beautiful thought from Gregory David Roberts, who wrote the extraordinary tale of his journey through India in his book *Shantaram*. This line from the end of his book again brings to mind the limitless possibilities that every single moment brings with it: 'Every human heartbeat is a universe of possibilities.'

NOTE on he or she.
I couldn't come to peace with which term to use, as both are of course equal. But I finally decided that as I have two beautiful sons I would honour the feminine—and the daughters I never gave birth to—and use 'she'. Admittedly this is not a very good reason but it is the only one I can come to rest with!

CHAPTER 1

UNDERSTANDING YOGA

The word *yoga* derives from the Sanskrit *yuj*, which means 'to join', 'to unify', 'coming together', 'oneness' or 'yoke'. The practice of yoga is a union of the whole person—the soul, the mind, the emotions and the physical body. It is a coming together of our human selves with the more divine aspects of our being—that is, our higher consciousness, our divinity, or the way we interpret God in our lives. When yoga is practised regularly, we develop a deeper and more profound understanding of the spiritual aspects of our nature, our physical bodies become more subtle and strong, and balance is established in the mental and emotional parts of our being.

Archaeological evidence suggests that yoga has been around for more than 10,000 years. Statues depicting yoga postures and meditation positions from

that time have been discovered in the Indus Valley in Pakistan. The *Vedas*, the first books on yoga, were written around that time and are most sacred books in Hindu literature. Included in the *Vedas* are the *Upanishads*, the philosophical part of the *Vedas*.

The first systemic writing on yoga was put together by the sage Patanjali. His text is called the *Yoga Sutras* and is still closely followed today. Patanjali's work is often referred to as the Eight-Fold Path, consisting of:

1. *Yama*—self-restraint
2. *Niyama*—self-observation
3. *Asana*—physical postures
4. *Pranayama*—breathing exercises
5. *Pratyahara*—becoming less associated with the outside world, withdrawal of the consciousness from the external environment
6. *Dharana*—concentration

7. *Dhyana*—meditation
8. *Samadi*—ultimate awareness of pure consciousness (B.K.S. Iyengar, *Light on Yoga*, page 3).

These eight aspects provide an excellent guide for any yoga practitioner, while being also one of the paths ascribed to for a better understanding of the self and ultimately to self-realisation.

Yoga is the control of the waves of the mind. Normally the self is identified with these waves, but it is possible to free it so that it rests on its own.
Patanjali, in Ronald Hutchinson, Yoga: A Way of Life

Hatha Yoga is the term most commonly used to describe the system of yoga that is taught today. In its truest form Hatha Yoga is a series of advanced cleansing techniques that are still practised, but usually only by very experienced yogis or those dedicated to yoga in its purest form. I will be dealing primarily with Hatha Yoga as we know it today.

Even when Hatha Yoga is taken up purely as a form of physical exercise, when the body becomes more agile, supple and relaxed the inner calmness experienced seems to overflow naturally to mental, emotional and spiritual aspects, positively affecting the whole person. Although these aspects of yoga can each be practised separately they are interconnected with each other and therefore influence the whole person, mind, body and spirit. For example, when a posture is being done with full breath and mind awareness the results are advantageous for the body as well as calming and centring the atmosphere of the mind. In the purest form every practice of yoga involves breath awareness—it is the foundation of the postures, of meditation and relaxation.

One of the traditional yogic teachings is *Tantra Yoga*, an in-depth study involving the spiritual *chakra* system. All yoga practices have a subtle influence on this spiritual element of yoga—the postures, breathing and meditation—whether the practitioner is interested in them or not. Chapter 14, Creative meditations and visualisation, includes a chakra meditation for pregnancy that most women thoroughly enjoy, using the specific colours from Tantra Yoga.

Briefly, there are seven major chakras, or energy centres, located within the spiritual body and symbolically situated along the inner side of the spinal column. The chakras are connected to each other by psychic channels called *nadis*, which are analogous to the network of nerves that connect to the central nervous system. In yogic teachings energy, or *prana*, flows through the psychic body along these nadis, in a similar way that the nerves in our bodies send energy via nerve impulses through our physical body and in Chinese philosophy energy or *chi* is carried along the meridians.

Corresponding to the spinal column in the spiritual sense is the most important nadi, known as *sushumna nadi*. There are 72,000 nadis, the main ones crossing each other at the chakra points along the spinal column.

When these systems are balanced, a person feels well and moves through life easily and in peace, but where there is an imbalance might begin to feel unwell, with physical problems emerging. This is also true in regard to the health of the emotions, which can be thrown out of balance because of the many stresses that are part of our daily lives. In Western health care systems there are various therapies and medicines for maintaining health in the nervous system while in traditional Chinese medicine acupuncture, herbal remedies and tai chi are used for creating health and wellbeing.

When the yoga postures are practised, even in their simplest forms, we are not only working on the physical body but gently stimulating and balancing our chakra system in the most subtle way. Every posture affects our physical, emotional and psychic bodies so that through practice harmony is established in the body, mind and spirit.

Through the ongoing practice of the ancient skills and teachings of yoga we have the opportunity to form a 'communion' with ourselves, to create a union with our entire nature, which allows us to embrace what yoga really means in its simplest yet purest form. This enables us to come together more as an individual, to merge our outer and inner selves more completely and to discover a peaceful, gentle place at the very centre of our beings. In pregnancy these concepts are gently incorporated into what I refer to as conscious birthing, a oneness of mind, body and soul—of woman, mother and child.

Yoga and Meditation for Pregnancy

Yoga for pregnancy has the same postures and breathing exercises found in general yoga and follows the same principles, but is approached in a very different way. It is designed specifically with the needs of the pregnant woman in mind, as the health and safety of mother and baby are the foremost, the most important, and only, consideration.

Always gentle, always replenishing, this form of yoga is as unique as is this time in a woman's life. It is about nourishing yourself as a pregnant woman and a mother, and being as one with your baby in your womb—ever mindful that you are pregnant and that your baby is a completely new soul with its own unique destiny and life path. Your yoga practice allows you to embrace that awareness and be present—as in a meditation, and to reflect on the constant transformation that is taking place in yourself and to marvel at the new life within you. This is what conscious birthing is about.

Practicing the different aspects of yoga is fulfilling and satisfying with unlimited benefits at every level of your being. You will feel well in your body and more relaxed in your emotions. Your awareness naturally increases during pregnancy and in time you become more insightful and intuitive. You will come to realise a deeper knowing and understanding through time spent in quiet reflection and contemplation, and look forward to time alone and at peace with yourself and with your baby. Most women who have enjoyed yoga while they were pregnant say they have a close bond with their babies when they are born and are in tune with them, and that their babies are calm and peaceful in their new life. Pregnancy is but a brief moment in your lifetime, it

is a precious opportunity to honour and nourish yourself as a pregnant woman and to be with your baby in the womb while preparing for the ultimate joy of life after birth.

A Balanced Yoga Program

A balanced yoga program includes the postures (*asanas*), yoga breathing exercises (*pranayama*), meditation (*dhyana*), the gestures (*mudras*) and deep relaxation (*yoga nidra*). During pregnancy a complete yoga program will nourish you in many ways and replenish your energies so you can enjoy this brief and wonderful time.

Benefits

The Postures: Asanas

The yoga exercises recommended are always gentle and generally easy to do; most of them can be modified so that you can enjoy them even if you are new to

yoga. They are safe to commence as soon as you have the okay from your health professionals and can be continued until full-term pregnancy, and even in the early moments of labour. A number of women have chosen to stay in class when they were in pre-labour and even when they were feeling the milder contractions of real labour. They trusted themselves and were relaxed enough to breathe gently through these first moments, feeling safe and supported in the company of other pregnant women. For them it was a gentle, calm way to embrace the earliest moments of their baby's journey from life in the womb to a new life in the world, an opportunity to reflect on a wondrous life experience before full labour was established.

Primarily, the asanas tone, strengthen and stretch your whole body while helping to release tightness, tension or stiffness in your muscles. They help you develop flexibility and suppleness as stretch and strength are equalised and

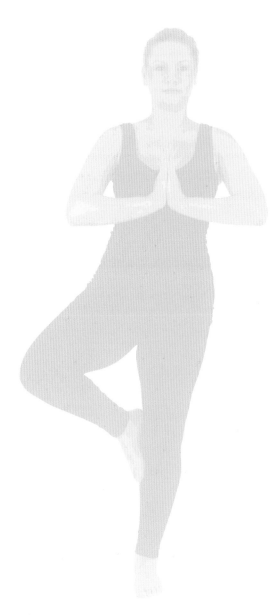

balanced on both sides of your body. The health of the nervous system is improved and harmonised, while the health of the endocrine glands, the function of the digestive system, and the fitness of the musculoskeletal system is also dramatically improved. Circulation is increased to all areas of the body and an enriched blood supply, combined with greater oxygen utilisation, has an overall nourishing effect. The end result is a much improved sense of wellbeing on a physical level, less fatigue, and enhanced emotional wellbeing. A number of the positions are also suitable to use during labour to overcome discomfort and for relaxation.

Of most significance are the benefits that yoga has for the female reproductive system. It provides a gentle and supportive health care program for both mother and baby during pregnancy which overflows into life after birth.

The postures are an effective way to help you overcome some of the more common physical discomforts that occur during pregnancy, and complement other therapies and health care choices. You will often need less alternative care and be able to better manage any discomforts yourself. When a posture is held, always be conscious of your breathing, how your body feels, where your thoughts are taking you and the atmosphere they create in your mind, so the posture is always safe, centring and quite beautiful to do. By practising yoga with complete body, breath and mind awareness you are fully conscious of the

moment and, in the process, observing the uniqueness and wonder of your whole body, mind and spirit. This is meditation within the postures.

The Breathing Exercises: Pranayama
Pranayama is not just deep breathing. It is a specific group of traditional yoga breathing exercises that are excellent to have knowledge of during pregnancy and especially during the birthing process. The asanas are obviously very important, but in many ways pranayama is even more important. These simple exercises benefit the health of the whole person and are what women rely on most, and feel empowered by, during the birthing process. Knowing how to breathe and breathe well, to use these techniques and trust the potential in the breath, is to breathe consciously and to birth consciously. Feeling confident in their breathing helps many women embrace their labour, often times with remarkable results. Breath awareness means you are totally present, where your attention is right there in the moment—not in the past and not in the future. Present moment awareness means you have clarity and insight, are steady and mindful, qualities that give you strength, courage and confidence. These qualities are precisely what a birthing woman needs knowledge of.

When we breathe more efficiently, oxygen utilisation and uptake are greatly improved. This life-giving oxygen reaches every cell so that your whole body is positively affected and recharged with energy, which is therapeutic for you and your baby. In yoga, this vital energy within the breath is known as *prana*, or the life force, and is carried with the breath through the body and mind. Correct breathing encourages deeper relaxation in your body and more peace in your mind, from where your meditation practice can naturally evolve. Bringing your attention to the natural breath is the foundation of all meditation practices and will prove an invaluable skill in pregnancy and in your life after the birth.

Meditation and Deep Relaxation

Meditation (*dhyana*) and deep relaxation (*yoga nidra*) are equally as important as the asanas and pranayama and should always be included in a pregnancy yoga class. These gentle practices allow you the time for inner reflection and quiet contemplation, to be mindful of the present, and provide a little peace and stillness in your day. The time spent in meditation or deep relaxation need only be 10 or 15 minutes, but the result is true rest and rejuvenation at all levels.

The correct body posture, ensuring greater body awareness, will help you gain the most from your time in meditation. To benefit from the healing potential in the breath you must first know how to breathe correctly, and understand what pranayama is, which will encourage relaxation and peace of mind. And to meditate you must first be able to relax. One cannot truly

exist without the other—this is yoga in its purest form.

Conscious birthing is about knowledge of breathing and the ability to relax deeply. They are what will help you the most during labour. When you are relaxed and following the flow of the breath as it moves through your body, you are there in your mind with your baby as you both progress through the contractions. Staying relaxed will have a significant influence on how your labour progresses and the atmosphere of this important day. You will feel strong, calm and confident. This will encourage you to trust in yourself, surrender to the process of birth and to accept what this birthday of your baby brings with it. Trust, surrender and accept.

The meditation practices are a very special part of pregnancy yoga, and many women say that it is this part of yoga they most enjoy. Meditation for pregnancy is both traditional and creative, with many benefits as a birth preparation, but especially that it takes you to a quiet peaceful place within yourself. These quieter moments provide you with the opportunity to just be with your baby, to come to know each other and to feel the love and bond between you before the birth. When you are relaxed the atmosphere in your womb will also be calm. Time in stillness is so nourishing for you as a woman and as a mother, and a special way for you to take care of you.

All aspects of yoga are valuable for promoting health and wellness, and when

these quieter aspects of yoga are used in conjunction with other therapies, many physical and emotional problems can be better managed and greatly improved over time.

When Should You Start Yoga?

As a general guide it is not recommended to commence the yoga postures until the second trimester (about 12 or 14 weeks) of pregnancy. Before this time I suggest you practise the yoga breathing exercises and meditation, and spend time just relaxing, focusing on the early days of being a mother and being there with your new baby. I do, however, recommend getting into the habit of doing the pelvic floor exercises, described on page 84, every day.

Many women experience fatigue and exhaustion in the early weeks of pregnancy; it is the body telling them to rest, to take time to relax. With all the changes taking place in your body it can take some time to recover your energies

> **NOTE:** If you don't start to feel better and the fatigue continues it would be a good idea to see your doctor. It could be that your iron levels are low or that your blood pressure is the reason for your persistent tiredness. Be constantly mindful of how you are feeling, never straining or pushing yourself if you don't feel well or are exhausted.

and rather than resisting the urge to sleep, it is better for you and your baby to give in and rest. The majority of women begin to feel better in the second trimester. It is not necessary to have practised yoga before conception, as pregnancy yoga is gentle and suitable for all women, of all fitness levels and all degrees of flexibility. Sometimes women don't start yoga until well into their pregnancies, but even yoga classes in the last few weeks are still worthwhile. Often the skills learnt during these few classes are enough to benefit them during labour.

Even though this form of yoga is very gentle it is important that you take responsibility for how you are feeling on a daily basis. The health and wellbeing of you and your baby are really the only things to consider. When you approach yoga in this way you will enjoy it more and reduce the risk of strain from over-effort. If you are attending regular classes, inform your teacher as soon as you become aware of your pregnancy and be certain that she is skilled in teaching pregnant women and aware of the precautions needed. A proper pregnancy yoga class is always safe, but it is still very important that you feel comfortable and secure, and confident in your teacher, at all times, and inform her of any concerns you have. Starting early in your second trimester helpful if you are not feeling very pregnant, as it brings the bond and closeness of mother and baby into your life early in your pregnancy. If you are

attending a pregnancy yoga class you will learn from the other women, share their experiences and enjoy the bond that naturally exists between pregnant women. Many women attending my classes have made lifelong friends and have found these connections a valuable support when their babies are born.

Pre-conception is also an important time in your life. If you are planning to conceive I suggest going to a few yoga classes to prepare your mind and body for pregnancy, being mindful that you are about to invite a precious new soul into your life.

Precautions

Yoga during pregnancy provides a gentle, safe and supportive health-care program for both mother and baby. It should always be gentle and relaxed where the wellbeing of you and the baby in your womb is the foremost consideration. Before you begin the exercises in this book or undertake any yoga class, always discuss your intentions with your doctor or midwife to ensure that yoga will be suitable for you, and to give you a feeling of confidence.

Choose a teacher who is experienced in teaching pregnant women and has a thorough understanding of pregnancy and what can be expected, physically and emotionally. At no time should you ever strain while doing the various postures, experience pain or discomfort. Every movement is to be enjoyed and relaxed

into so that you feel its benefits. You might notice a little tightness in your muscles when you first start, especially if you have not been doing some other form of stretching exercises. Even if you are very fit, take care when you begin yoga.

If you have had a miscarriage in the past, if you have a history of threatened miscarriages or if you have any concerns about your pregnancy, do not begin the physical exercises until after the fourth month of pregnancy. The breathing exercises, meditation and relaxation practices can be commenced as soon as possible after conception. If you have a disability or a delicate health condition, always consult a skilled yoga teacher so that the practices can be modified to suit your needs.

The physical exercises I recommend are specific for pregnant women. They can assist throughout the pregnancy by increasing physical tone and strength for a feeling of complete wellness. They are designed to work specifically on the parts of your body most involved in pregnancy and to allow optimum organ function and health. As the days draw closer to the birth you might need to adjust what you do and how you do it, and if need be leave a few of the postures out completely. Nearly all the exercises here can easily be modified so that you can continue with most of them until labour begins. Discontinue a posture immediately if you feel faint, light-headed, dizzy or nauseous. If you are tired, spend time doing the

CAUTION: If you have high or low blood pressure avoid all head-down postures and follow the modifications recommended. Even if your blood pressure is normal, always return to the standing position very slowly, for example taking two breaths to return to the standing position. If you have varicose veins or swollen feet avoid all postures where you are sitting on your feet and follow the modifications recommended for squatting.

yoga breathing and meditation or in deep relaxation instead of the exercises; they will quickly help restore your energies.

If you have lower back problems and sciatica you will find the postures are an excellent way to ease your discomfort as your pregnancy progresses. If you are having physiotherapy or other treatment, always ask your therapist's advice as to what you can and cannot do, and pass this on your yoga teacher. Most of the exercises can be modified to enable you to continue, but only if you are comfortable and able to relax completely into the pose.

To come onto your back from a seated position turn to the side and using your hands for support lower yourself to the floor and then roll onto your back. Always rest with your knees bent. To return to a seated position, roll onto your side and use your hands to push yourself up. This

procedure should also be used when lying down and sitting up in bed to reduce strain on your lower back and abdominal muscles.

If your baby is in the posterior position, it is helpful to sit in a more forward position rather than leaning back, especially from 30 weeks onward. Leaning forward encourages your baby to come into the optimum anterior position for birth. Spending time on the hands and knees doing pelvic rocking, the Cat or the Child Pose, especially with the hips elevated, will often help your baby to change position. This is also relevant if your baby is breech, although this is a more challenging position to change. In both of these situations always talk to your baby in quiet meditation and ask her to move—but, importantly, only if it is safe for you, and her to do so. Sometimes there is an internal reason why a baby is in one

of these positions. A full squatting position is not recommended if your baby is either posterior or breech—instead, squat on a stool or an exercise ball where your knees are in line with your hips, or even a little higher. This is because the pelvis is considerably wider in a full squat and can encourage the baby to descend and engage for birth—which is ideal if she is in the correct position, but not if she is in the wrong one.

What You Will Need

Very little equipment is required to enjoy your yoga time and no great cost need be incurred. Wear loose comfortable clothing that is not restricting around the waist and chest. No shoes are required. Two or three firm cushions are a good idea for support and comfort, and a rubber exercise mat the length of your body is desirable if the floor is hard and cold.

CAUTION: Some women feel uncomfortable lying on their back as early as the first trimester, but generally this occurs around 15–20 weeks when it is suggested you rest on your side instead. (It is usually recommended you rest on your left side but either side is acceptable.) The discomfort is due to pressure from the weight of the abdomen on the vena cava, a major vein on the right side of the body. Although it isn't dangerous to lie on your back, it can cause nausea and backache, especially in the last trimester. If you want to rest on your back always put a cushion under your head, another under the right hip to take the pressure away from your right side, and bend your knees. Using cushions is often enough to relieve any discomfort, but if not rest on your side in the Flapping Fish Pose (see page 147). (This is useful information if you need to lie on your back for some time for a medical procedure.)

I highly recommend a bean bag for comfort while sitting for the breathing exercises and meditations, for use while practising some of the postures, and as a great birthing aid. Many women enjoy their bean bags so much that if the hospital doesn't provide them they take their own to the birth. Fill the bean bag with two or two and a half bags of beans rather than the recommended three; this gives more flexibility and greater comfort.

A low stool is another great idea, especially for the squatting exercises. It will also be useful in the standing forward-bending postures, as you can lean on the stool rather than resting your hands on your legs or the floor. If you have high or low blood pressure and don't want to have your head down, resting your hands on the stool and looking straight ahead is a suitable alternative. If your baby is in the posterior position, leaning forward on the stool from a seated, squatting or standing position is recommended to encourage her to turn into the anterior position. An exercise ball is also useful; a number of the exercises can be practised on one, while it is a valuable asset during labour.

Practise your yoga in a room free of draughts or direct sunlight and move any furniture that may hinder your movements. In the hotter weather drink plenty of water to prevent dehydration. During the cooler months, cover your body with a blanket when you are in the resting positions and wear socks because your body temperature will drop when you relax and your feet are the first part of your body to feel cool.

Generally, yoga is practised when the bowels and bladder are empty, and at least three hours after a meal, but this is not always possible during pregnancy. If you have a problem with hypoglycaemia or diabetes, eat a small amount of food beforehand and, if need be, snack on dry biscuits or nuts during the class.

How Often Should You Practise?

It is a personal choice how often you practise yoga and meditation, as it will depend on how much time you have available and how you are feeling. You will know better than anybody else what is best for you and it is important to go with your instincts. Some women attend a class once a week and feel this is both sufficient and beneficial, others like to practise more regularly, either in a class or at home. Always listen to your own intuition about how much to do and how often to practise—sometimes you might just want to do the yoga postures, especially if you have physical problems which these movements often relieve. At other times you might prefer to concentrate on the breathing exercises and meditations, especially if you are tired. Every woman will approach her pregnancy and her yoga in a different way. The practices and suggestions are there for you to follow at your own pace to ensure you have a happy and healthy pregnancy.

CHAPTER 2

WARMING UP:
FLOOR EXERCISES AND POSTURES

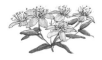

You are where your attention takes you. In fact, you are your attention. If your attention is fragmented, you are fragmented. When your attention is in the past, you are in the past. When your attention is in the present moment, you are in the presence of God and God is present in you.

Deepak Chopra, *Creating Affluence,*
page 61

These warming-up exercises and gentle yoga postures are an excellent way to tone and loosen your body before practising the other asanas. They can also be practised on their own as a complete floor program and are especially useful if you are feeling tired or if your doctor has suggested a lighter yoga program.

Before commencing your yoga I suggest you spend a little time with your awareness on your breathing to centre and your mind and calm your emotions (see chapter 11, Breathing exercises: pranayama, page 95). This will help relax your body in preparation for the exercises,

bring your awareness to the atmosphere of your mind and your attention into the present moment.

Exercises for the Feet and Ankles

These very simple exercises are recommended before practising any of the other seated postures and the squatting exercises. They are an excellent way to loosen the ankles and increase flexibility in the feet and can help to relieve fluid retention, especially in the last weeks of pregnancy.

1. Sit on the floor with the legs straight in front of you. For comfort you can sit against the wall or on cushions. Rest your hands behind your back for extra support and comfort.

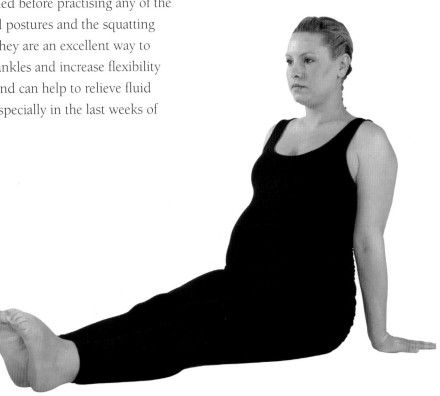

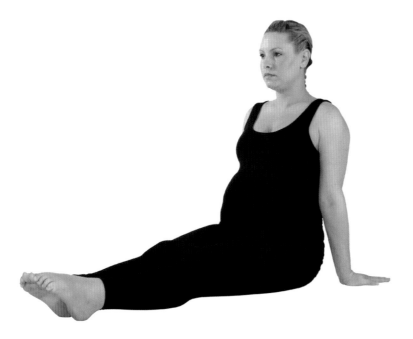

2. Point the toes down and feel the stretch in the tops of the feet.

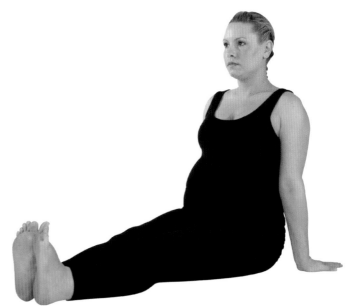

3. Flex the feet up. Do these movements slowly so that you feel a deep stretch into the lower legs as well. This can be repeated five times.

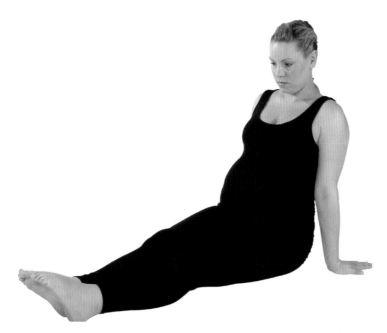

4. Make big slow circles with the feet, five times to the right and five times to the left.

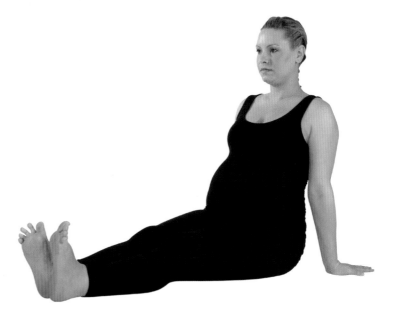

5. Spread the toes wide apart, then squeeze them tightly together. Repeat this three times.

Hip Rotations: *Shoni Chakra*

The Hip Rotations are an important exercise for pregnancy and can be used as a preparation for postures that involve the hips, such as the Butterfly, Squatting, and the Wide-A Leg Stretches. This exercise will tone and open your pelvic area, while giving increased flexibility and freedom of movement to your hips. It might feel quite awkward to begin with, but if you concentrate on making large circles with your knee, rather than with your hip, you will find it less difficult. Always approach it slowly, making big circles in both directions.

1. Sit on the floor, or on cushions, with your spine straight and your legs in front of you.

2. Bend your left leg. Hold onto your left foot with your right hand and your left knee with your left hand.

3. Make slow circles with the left knee so as to rotate your whole hip. Repeat this five times in a clockwise direction and five times in an anticlockwise direction. Shake your leg lightly when you have completed the exercise.

4. Repeat the exercise rotating your right hip.

The Half Butterfly

The Half Butterfly is an excellent way to prepare for the Butterfly and other postures where flexibility is required in your hip and inner thigh areas.

1. Sit on the floor with your back straight and relaxed. Your right leg is straight and your left knee is bent. Rest your left foot on top of your right thigh or, if this is not comfortable, place the sole of your left foot beside your right thigh. Your ankle needs to be quite supple before your foot can comfortably be placed on top of your thigh, but with regular practice of the exercises for your feet and the hip rotations, greater flexibility will be achieved over time.

2. Hold onto your foot and your knee and bounce your left leg freely up and down without straining. Practise this movement nine times before changing legs and repeating it with your right leg.

Some women are naturally very flexible in the hip and inner thigh areas and will find these practices much easier than other women do. Don't worry if your knee doesn't reach the floor when you first begin, for with time you will become more open and supple.

The Butterfly: *Baddhakonasana*

The Butterfly is one of the most important seated positions to consider as an antenatal exercise. Your whole pelvic region, your inner thighs and your hips are 'opened' and toned, without any stress being applied. The abductor muscles of your inner thigh are stretched and strengthened. The Butterfly improves

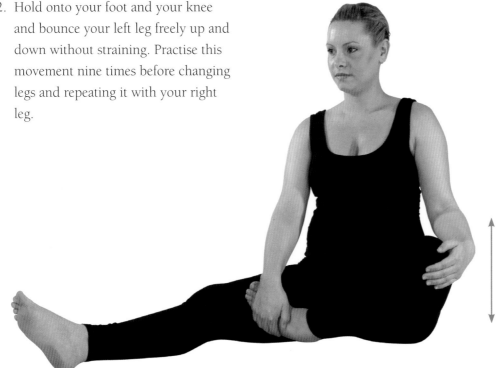

circulation as well as kidney and bladder function. Your reproductive system is balanced, establishing excellent organ function and integrity. Women who sit in this posture regularly often have an easier delivery and recovery after the birth, as is also the case with the Squatting exercises.

It is very important not to force your knees towards the floor or strain yourself in any way; their movement should always be gentle and relaxed. When you first practise the Butterfly, spend some time sitting with the soles of your feet together. If you are tight in the inner thigh area, sit with your back against a wall for extra support and, if need be, use a small cushion. Cushions can also be placed under your knees for support; when your flexibility increases they can be removed.

Variation 1

1. Sit with your back straight and relaxed, the soles of your feet together and your hands holding onto your feet. If you feel the stretch is too strong, place a cushion under each knee. If you lean slightly back from the upright position your knees will naturally come closer to the floor and you will not have to apply any downward pressure.

2. With gentle movements, move your knees up and down like a butterfly's wings, remembering not to force them towards the floor. The object of this exercise is to open and stretch your inner thigh and pelvic area without

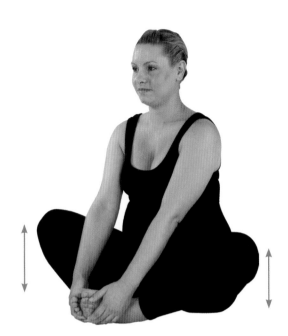

forcing your legs onto the floor. Many women are initially quite stiff when attempting this exercise, but with a little patience and regular practice their flexibility soon improves.

To increase your flexibility, the Butterfly posture can be practised lying on your back—without the movements—either on the floor or on a bed. (Remember to follow the guides for resting on your back.) If you find this is comfortable, you can use it for resting and relaxing. The effects of gravity are greater when lying on your back and your knees will naturally fall towards the floor. As there is virtually

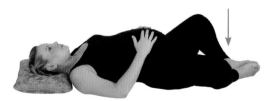

no pressure on your back in this position, it is better for those who have a weak lower back or back pain during the last trimester. Again, cushions can be placed under your knees. This variation can also be practised with the legs resting up against the wall as detailed in the chapter Squatting (see page 55).

Variation 2

1. From the seated Butterfly posture, breathe in as you ease your knees towards the floor while lifting up your feet with your hands. Straighten your back and look up.
2. Breathe out and bring your head toward your feet. Press your elbows lightly into your calf muscles or lower legs as your knees are eased towards the floor. Keep your shoulders relaxed at all times.
3. Repeat these two movements up to five times, breathing in and out rhythmically as you move from position 1 to position 2. When you inhale, try to straighten your back and stretch fully through your spinal column, feeling the upward lift of your body, and the opposite sensation in your legs as you bend over and your knees are pressed to the floor. As an alternative, hold the forward bending position for three or four breaths to benefit more from the inner thigh stretch, always remembering to keep the shoulders and arms relaxed as you hold the position.

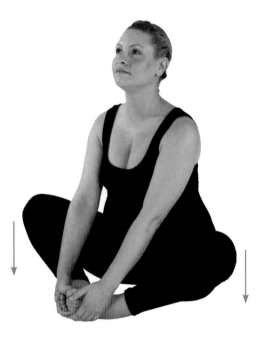

4. On completion extend your legs slightly forward and relax into the Sleeping Tortoise (page 148).

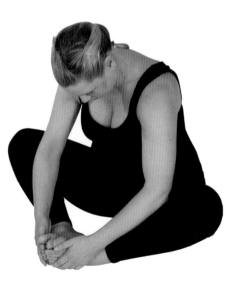

Note: Before commencing the next group of exercises it is important to have loosened your body with the previous group. This way you will not be at risk of injury due to cold and tight muscles, and you will benefit more. Keep in mind that there is never any need to compare yourself with others or to find fault in your own achievements—just remember to relax and enjoy your yoga. When yoga is approached in a rigid manner, you are likely to find yourself becoming stiff or sore.

The Equestrian Pose: *Ashwa Sanchalanasana*

`The four previous poses provide an ideal warm-up for the Equestrian pose, which is included among the seated postures because it is commenced from the knees.

This strong posture has excellent benefits for the pelvis, the hips and the lower back. I recommend placing a small cushion under your knee to protect your kneecap, especially if you have had a knee injury or if the floor is very hard. Although this is quite strong, most pregnant women enjoy the deep stretch in the inner thigh area and through the hip. It can be easily modified to achieve the best results and in comfort.

1. Commence from a kneeling position. Place your right foot flat on the floor with your right leg far enough forward to feel balanced and steady in this posture. A cushion can be placed under the left knee.

2. Place both hands on the inside of your right foot and move forward as far as you can in complete comfort so that your left leg is extended and stretched back. From this posture you will feel a deep expansion throughout your thigh, hip and pelvis. If your right heel comes away from the floor while lunging forward, your foot needs to be placed further forward before you begin, or maybe you are lunging too far forward.

3. Relax into the posture and hold it for five breaths or for as long as you are comfortable. When you first practise this I recommend you hold the final positions for only two or three breaths to avoid strain or discomfort. It is important to be relaxed and never strain as you move into the full stretch.

4. Inhale as you return to the upright position. You might like to relax into the Child Pose before changing sides.

5. Repeat with the left leg to the front.

6. Relax into the Child Pose to finish.

The Seated Triangle: *Pavishtha Konasana*

Also known as the Wide Leg Stretch, this is one of the most important exercises to practise regularly. As your pregnancy progresses, you will notice your body becoming looser and more supple due to the increase of relaxing hormones. This makes the wide leg stretches easier and more pleasurable to practise.

Always remember not to push yourself into the full posture or to over-extend, as it is easy to injure yourself this way. Spend a little extra time, using your breath and your awareness to ease and extend into the posture, staying as relaxed as possible to prevent tension building up in your body.

To relieve strain in your lower back—and for extra support—rest your lower back against a wall. You can also place a small cushion under your buttocks to slightly elevate your pelvis and tilt it forward.

In the wide leg stretches, the inner thigh muscles receive a deep full stretch, toning the muscles of your inner thigh and pelvis. The function of the whole pelvic region and the corresponding organs is greatly improved. These exercises have special advantages for pregnant women, even if you only spend time in the upright seated position.

When your body is stretched forward between your legs, the whole of your back is stretched, especially across the lower back and hips, and your abdomen and pelvis are gently compressed and massaged.

When the stretch is taken over the right and left legs, the organs of digestion are stimulated and the spinal nerves benefit from a renewed blood flow. Also, as your head is down in the forward bend and side stretches, your mind becomes quiet and calm, giving you the opportunity to breathe and relax into the posture. Even though it might not feel like a relaxation pose initially, when time is spent in the forward stretch your mind will become quiet and peaceful. This is a fine example of when yoga is approached in a calm and gentle way the postures become a meditation within the movement.

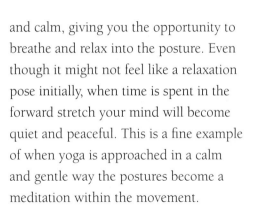

> Note: The Wide Leg Stretch is another exercise that can be practised lying on your back with your legs up against a wall. I mention this because some women find it difficult sitting in this position with their backs straight, or have back and hip problems which make it unsuitable. Women who develop lower back problems or sciatica during the later part of pregnancy should also practise it with their legs up a wall. See page 55 for full details. For women who are carrying high or who are short in the body, the forward bending position might become uncomfortable in the last trimester. In this case, stretch gently to the side.

The greatest benefits are received from all the forward bending postures when the final position is held for an extended period, allowing the body plenty of time to relax into the stretch. This gives the associated muscles the opportunity to adjust and extend gradually and gently.

When you first sit in the wide leg stretch, spend some time flexing your feet and pointing your toes to stretch your calf muscles and loosen your ankles.

Stretching Forward

1. Sit with your legs as wide apart as possible, your spine straight and your shoulders relaxed. Breathe in and feel as if you are lifting your body upwards from the base of your spine.
2. Breathe out as you bend forward from your waist. Keep your shoulders and arms loose and relaxed and your

> **Note:** When this group of seated postures is completed it is important to practise a suitable counter-pose to relieve any discomfort in your back. You can either lie on your back and bring your knees into your chest, gently rocking your body from side to side, or practise the Pelvic Tilt (page 43), Pelvic Rocking on the hands and knees (page 37), the Child Pose (page 63) or the Cat (page 40).

elbows slightly bent to prevent tension being held in your shoulders and upper back. Rest your hands on the floor in front of you and relax your head and neck. Holding the posture, release any tightness in your body and breathe quietly into the stretch. At no time strain or force yourself forward but use your breathing and your awareness to ease as far into the posture as possible. The more time you spend breathing into the posture and concentrating on releasing tightness and discomfort, the deeper you will go

and the more relaxed you are going to feel.

Some women are able to stretch forward easily, able to rest elbows and head on the floor even at full-term pregnancy. Others can stretch forward only a little. How far you move forward is not the main focus in this pose. It is your overall approach that is important—how you are feeling in your body, where your thoughts are at the time, that your awareness is on breathing in a steady and relaxed manner. We are all different—some of us are very supple and have great freedom of movement, others are tighter in the body and have less flexibility. Some women enjoy this posture more with a bean bag between their legs to lean over onto. In this way they are supported and can really rest and relax into the pose. A bean bag is especially useful if you have a lower back problem, pelvic discomfort or pelvic instability.

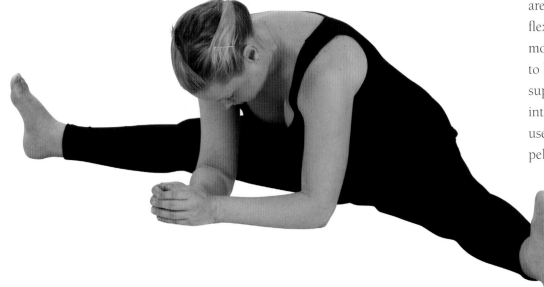

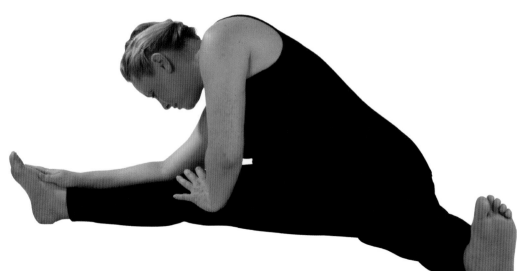

Churning the Mill: *Chakki Chahalasana*

This exercise has been modified for pregnancy. Some women find the gentle movement from one side to the other a little easier to do than the stronger forward or side bends of the Wide Leg Stretch.

The same benefits are derived from this exercise, with the bonus that as your body moves freely from the left to the right your waist is also toned. With practice, your hips and spine will become looser and more flexible. Tension is relieved in your shoulders and upper back due to the position of your arms.

Stretching Over Each Leg

1. From the wide leg position turn your body to the right. Breathe in and as you breathe out stretch your body over your right leg. Rest your hands on your leg with your arms slightly bent and bring your head down towards your knee. Take special care that your arms and shoulders are very relaxed. Only come forward to a position where you can hold the posture in a relaxed manner and without bending your knee. Feel the deep stretch throughout your back, in the side of your body and in the hamstrings and thigh muscles. If there is any strain or discomfort, ease out of the posture slightly. Hold the final posture for five breaths.

3. Breathe in as you return to the seated position. Repeat the posture, stretching over your left leg. Depending on your stage of pregnancy and where your baby is lying, you will usually find that one side is a lot easier to do than the other.

1. Sit with your back straight and legs as wide apart as possible. For extra comfort place a small cushion under your buttocks. Lift your arms to the centre front at shoulder height and join your hands together with interlocking fingers.

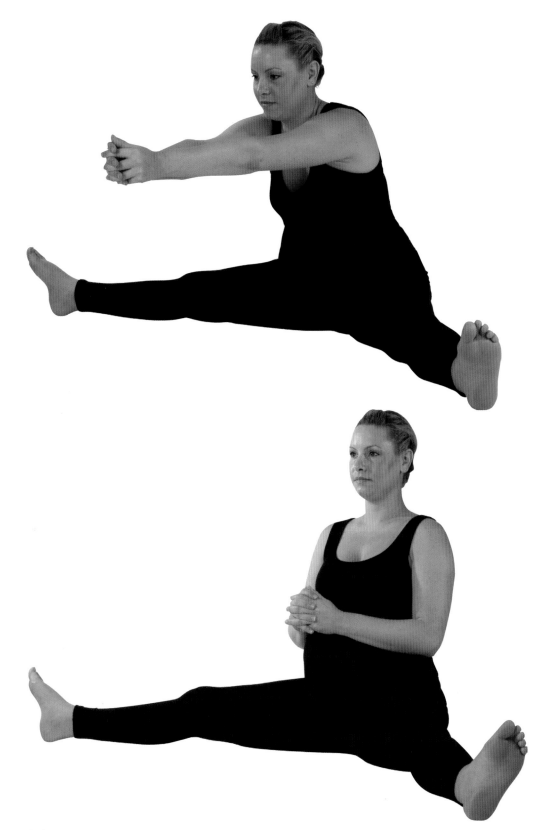

2. Lean slightly forward and then move your body slowly to the right while breathing in.

3. Breathe out as you move your body to the left. The idea is to create a slow, sweeping semi-circular movement, moving continuously from right to left. Repeat this five times to each side.

4. Continue with this movement and as you inhale lean slightly back, bending your arms and bringing your hands close into the body. Exhale as you lean forward, stretching as far forward as is comfortable, so that you are doing big slow circular movements. Repeat this five times to the right and five times to the left.

5. Bring your legs together when you have completed the posture and shake them lightly.

Working in Pairs

Working with a partner in the wide leg stretch is a very enjoyable way to practise this posture; some women prefer it to stretching alone. This variation enables you and your partner to move into the stretch more fully and to relax more deeply as it encourages less resistance and a deeper stretch through the back and inner thigh. It can be quite an effort to stretch forward alone but when working with a partner she eases you very gently into the forward position and vice versa. This means you will probably stretch further and, importantly, relax more in body and mind.

Choose a partner with a similar level of flexibility and about the same height. Sit with your legs as wide as possible, with your feet together and your hands joined. If you are more flexible than your partner, or have longer legs, ask her to place her feet on the inside of your ankles so that you both have your legs as wide as possible and will receive the maximum from the posture. Working together is meant to be easy and very relaxing, and because of this you will probably extend

further into the stretch. Communicate with each other throughout to ensure there is no risk of over-extension or strain. If the stretch is intense you have extended too far and should always ease out of the pose until you reach a comfortable stretch you can relax into.

Bending Forward

1. Sit on the floor with your partner with your legs as wide apart as is comfortable for both of you. Join your feet together and hold hands. At this point any necessary adjustments can be made to your positions.
2. Lean back slightly and gently ease your partner into the forward bending position. You must feel comfortable at all times and keep communicating with each other so that you are fully

aware of how far to move forward into the stretch. When your partner is in the forward stretch check that she is completely relaxed through her arms and shoulders, and she is breathing quietly into the posture. The more emphasis placed on breathing into the stretch, the more beneficial and the more relaxing it will be. At no time should either of you over-extend yourselves or move beyond a comfortable stretch. The point of this exercise is to have a sense of freedom and ease as you bend forward from your waist.
3. Remain in the forward stretch for five breaths before changing roles so that your partner stretches you forward.
4. Repeat this exercise three times each.

Note: If your partner is extremely flexible, hold her by the lower arms or elbows so you don't have to lean too far back; if you are both very flexible, sit a little further apart to allow the space to bend forward.

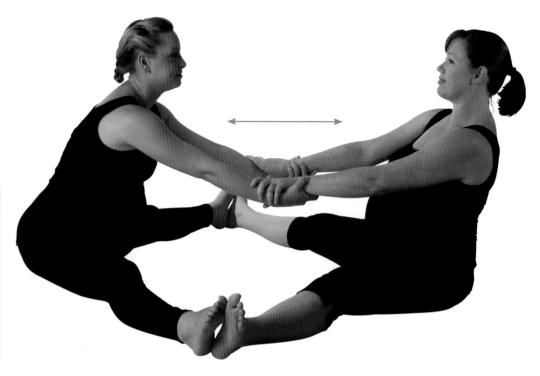

Slow Circles

This exercise greatly benefits the waist, hips, back, abdominal area and inner thighs. It is very similar to Churning the Mill (see below), except that in working with a partner more movement is involved in making complete circles.

1. From the same wide leg position, make slow wide circles with each other, gently leaning back, moving to one side, into the forward stretch and then moving to the other side. Make the circles slow and flowing.

2. Continue making slow full circles, five to the right and five to the left. Try to synchronise the movements with your breathing, so that you breathe out as you move forward and breathe in as you move back.

There seems to be a tendency to speed up when practising these circles, so be conscious of moving slowly. I am sure you will enjoy it much more when it is taken quietly.

On completion rest in the Child Pose or rest on your back and bring your knees into your body, rocking slowly from side to side.

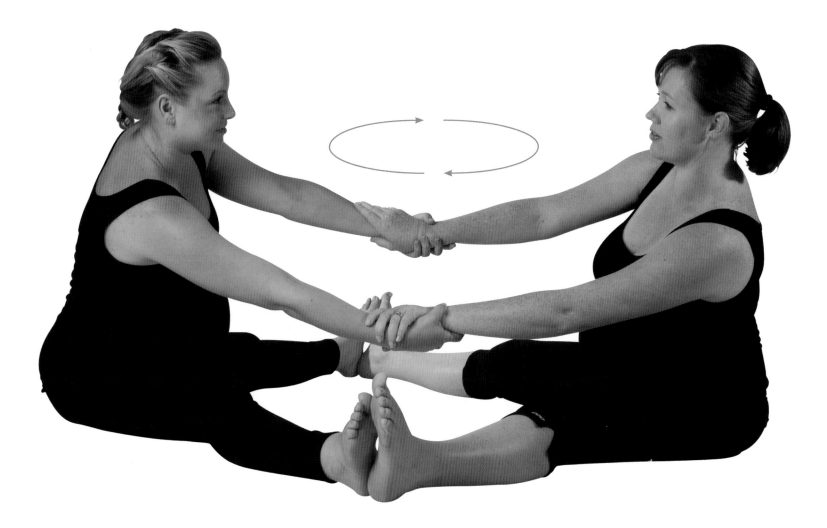

Pelvic Rocking

This is a lovely relaxing way to relieve discomfort in the pelvic area. It is excellent when there is a lower back problem or sciatica, and also recommended if your baby is not in the correct position for birth. It is ideally practised after the seated wide leg stretches, the Cat and the Tiger (pages 40 and 42). From the hands and knees position, simply make big wide circles with your hips, stretching back as far as you can to feel the wonderful stretch along the length of your spine, and then come forward to feel the weight on your hands, making it an ideal choice if you have swollen hands or carpal tunnel syndrome. In the forward position keep the hips level rather than dropping them downward, and be aware that the abdominal muscles are relaxed. The movements are slow and full and can be repeated as many times as you wish. Rest in the Child Pose on completion.

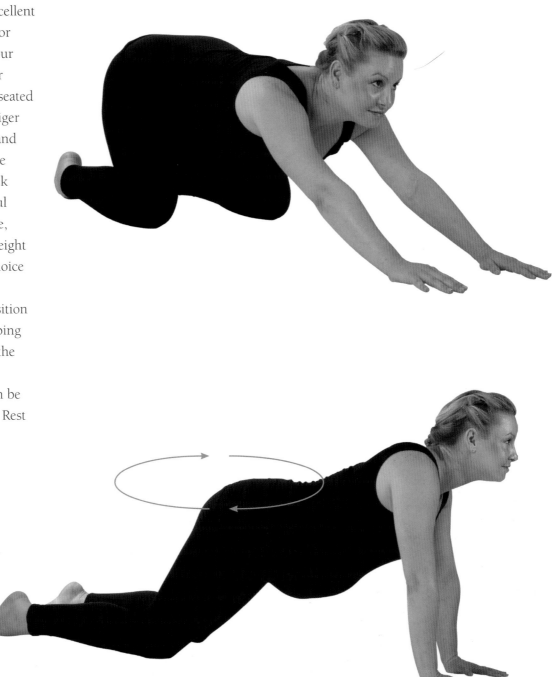

The Thunderbolt Pose: *Vajrasana*

The Thunderbolt or Diamond posture is used by many cultures. It is a favoured posture among Japanese Buddhists for meditation and prayer. It is a very comfortable posture to use for resting and quietening your mind, for practising pranayama, and during meditation. It is especially good in conjunction with the Breath Balancing pose (see page 94).

I suggest placing one or two small cushions between buttocks and heels to relieve any discomfort in your feet. A thin piece of foam padding can be placed under feet and ankles until they become accustomed to your weight resting on them.

The Thunderbolt posture improves circulation in your pelvic and other internal organs while your pelvic floor muscles are also strengthened. It is probably one of the most beneficial positions after a meal because your spine is straight and the digestive processes can function more efficiently. This is very important during pregnancy, when many women suffer from indigestion, and especially for those with peptic ulcers, hyperacidity, heartburn and bloating after eating. Your ankles and the muscles of your feet are stretched and loosened, helping relieve arthritis in your hips and your knees. When this position is first practised, remain there for a short time only to avoid unnecessary discomfort in your feet and ankles.

1. Sit in a kneeling position with your knees together, your big toes touching and your heels apart. Your back is relaxed and your spine is straight.

2. Rest the palms of your hands face-down on top of your thighs, or palms up in *bhairava mudra* (page 89) with one hand on top of the other, or use the Breath Balancing pose. This posture can be held for as long as you are comfortable.

> **Note:** The Thunderbolt pose is not recommended if you have varicose veins or swollen feet.

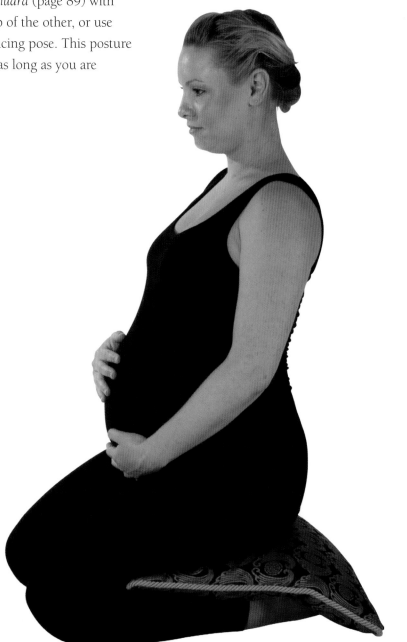

The Frog (with arm exercises): *Mandukasana*

The Frog is an excellent seated posture both for pregnancy and after the birth. It has all the benefits of the previous posture as well as stretching deeply into your inner thigh muscles due to the wide position of your legs. It is very useful for relieving tension throughout your hips, pelvic floor and whole pelvic and abdominal region, being especially important to the health of the female reproductive system and bladder.

These arm exercises are among the few where the muscles of your upper arms are toned, firmed and strengthened. However, if you find the Frog uncomfortable to hold, it is not necessary to do the arm exercises from this position. Any seated position where your back is straight and relaxed is also suitable, including sitting on a stool or in a chair.

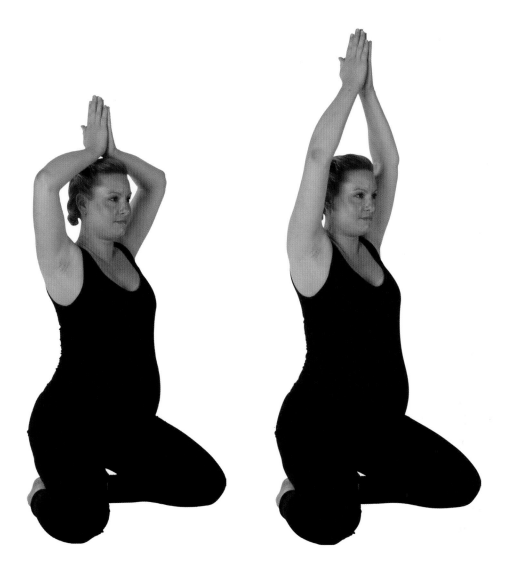

1. Kneel in the Thunderbolt posture, buttocks on heels and your big toes crossed or touching. Widen your knees as far as possible. One or two cushions can be placed under your buttocks for extra comfort. Feel your whole body relax into the posture.

2. Take your arms up above your head. Join your palms together and rest the heels of your hands on the crown of your head. Your shoulders stay down and relaxed throughout the exercise.

3. Breathe in as you raise and straighten your arms above your head while pressing the palms of your hands firmly together. If you push too hard you will cause strain and tension in your upper arms and shoulders.

4. Breathe out as the heels of your hands are lowered to the top of your head, again pressing the hands firmly together.

5. Repeat this as many times as you like, being aware of the strong sensations in your upper arms and chest. Done correctly, the Frog is quite a strenuous posture, requiring strength in your upper arms and shoulders. I usually suggest repeating it five or six times.

6. When you have completed the exercise, lower your arms and lightly shake your arms and hands. Stretch your legs out in front of you, shaking them lightly to restore the circulation and remove any stiffness.

The Head of the Cow: *Gomukhasana*

The Head of the Cow is another ideal exercise for your arms and shoulders and I recommend practising it regularly to maintain flexibility. It can be done from any seated position where your back is straight and relaxed, or while standing. You might notice it is much easier to do on one side than the other, but with regular practice both sides will eventually be the same. *Gomukhasana* refers to two things: *go* means 'cow' and *mukha* is 'face', indicating the face of a cow; while a

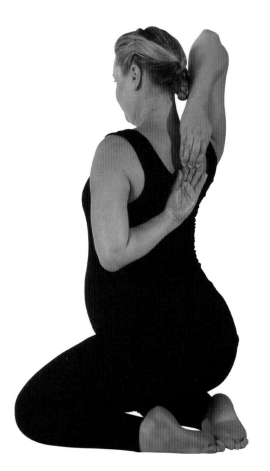

gomukha is a musical instrument that is broad at one end and narrow at the other, like a cow's face.

This posture works deeply into your shoulders, upper arms and neck muscles. It is very useful for relieving tension and inflexibility in these areas, and helpful for the relief of backache.

1. From a seated position bend your left arm up behind your back, taking your hand as high up the centre of your back as is comfortable.
2. Raise your right arm above your head and then take it over your right shoulder towards the fingers of your left hand, joining your fingers if possible. Hold your right arm in an upright position so that your elbow is pointing straight up and your upper arm is beside your ear. If you find that your fingers don't meet, a piece of rope or maybe a wooden spoon can be used to fill the gap until your fingers touch.
3. Once your fingers are together or joined otherwise, relax your shoulders and arms and breathe naturally. Remain in this position until you feel increasing warmth in your upper arm.
4. Lower your arms and shake them a little before repeating the exercise with your right arm up the middle of your back. I suggest this exercise be done twice as it is always a little easier the second time around.

The Cat: *Marjariasana*

The Cat is one of the most important postures to practise throughout pregnancy, with only a slight variation from the traditional form. The all fours position is particularly comfortable, as the weight taken away from your pelvic region relieves that heavy feeling often felt during the last trimester. Many women find the hands and knees position is very comfortable for contractions, especially if the baby is in the posterior position. If you use the Cat during labour it is ideal to relax into the Child Pose between contractions to rest and restore energy.

The Cat is especially good for your back, abdomen and pelvis. Lower back pain and stiffness are relieved as the Cat exercises your spine all the way from the neck through to the tail bone. Your pelvis is rocked forward and back, which tones the muscles and ligaments and works deeply into your reproductive system. Your whole internal body is toned and your uterine muscles gently massaged by the alternating movements.

It is useful if you suffer from groin pain in the last weeks before delivery, as weight is taken away from that area. The all fours position encourages deep breathing which ensures a good oxygen flow to your whole body, and is recommended if you have swollen hands or carpal tunnel syndrome. The Cat and the Tiger can be followed with pelvic rocking on hands and knees (page 37) and then resting in the Child Pose.

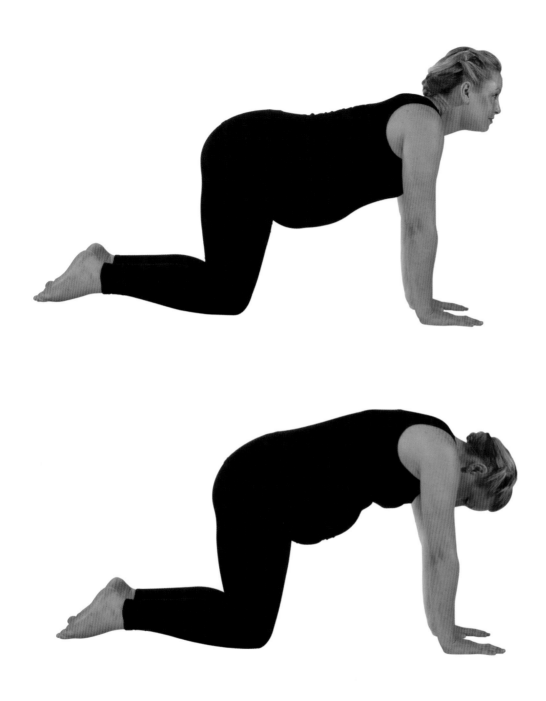

Also, in position 2 where your back is arched upwards, it is not recommended to contract your abdominal muscles while exhaling, but to keep these muscles relaxed. By practising the Cat gently and slowly, your whole spinal column and pelvic area will be massaged, toned and made wonderfully flexible.

1. Come into the all fours position, arms straight, with your knees the same distance apart as your hands and shoulders.
2. Hold your back straight and breathe in, looking straight ahead.
3. Breathe out as you arch your spine so your tail bone is tucked under and your chin comes close into your chest, remembering to keep your arms straight throughout the exercise.
4. Breathe in as you straighten your back. Repeat these movements five times, then relax into the Child Pose with your knees wide.

Caution: Because of the extra weight in your abdomen, it is important not to hollow your back in position 1 (as is done in the traditional pose). Keep your back straight when inhaling to lessen any strain on the ligaments, especially in the third trimester.

Caution: If you have pelvic pain or any instability in that area I do not recommend the Tiger.

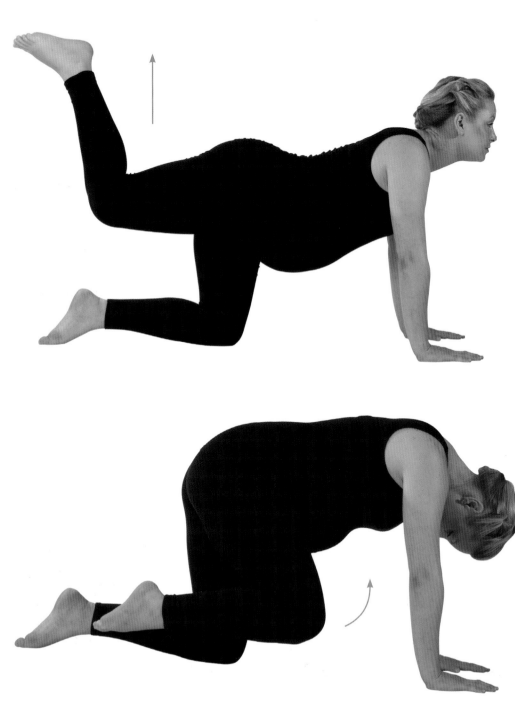

The Tiger: *Vyaghrasana*

The Tiger is similar to the Cat and usually follows on from it. The benefits are comparable, except that in the Tiger you receive an added stretch in your hip and lower back by extending your leg upward. This is an ideal exercise for the relief of lower back discomfort, and particularly sciatic pain as the leg is brought forward. Some people find the Tiger more strenuous than other exercises, so take care not to go beyond your level of fitness. From three and five movements on each side will work sufficiently into your hip and your leg.

1. From the all fours position, arms straight, breathe in as you raise your right leg behind you as high as possible. Lift your head slightly and look up. Some people like to straighten their leg in this elevated position but it can also stay slightly bent.

2. Breathe out as you bend your knee, bringing it underneath your body toward your face. Your back will be arched as in the Cat posture, and you will notice a gentle compression in your abdominal area.

3. Breathe in to lift your right leg again and repeat this up to five times. Shake your hands lightly and rest if you need to before repeating the movement five times with your left leg.

4. When you have completed each side, do some slow pelvic rocking and then relax into the Child Pose.

When you have completed the Cat and the Tiger I suggest spending some quite time relaxing into your favourite form of the Child Pose. A pleasant variation is to slightly elevate the hips, remembering to keep the back straight. This elevated position gives wonderful relief to the lower back and pelvic areas as well as having a deeply relaxing effect on the mind. You can remain in this for as long as you wish,

> **Caution:** Do not use this variation if you feel uncomfortable or are experiencing any fullness in the face, nor I do recommend it if you have high or low blood pressure.

but because your head has been lower than your heart, never sit up quickly; always rest with your head on your hands or in your hands before sitting up.

The Pelvic Tilt

The Pelvic Tilt is a modified version of the Shoulder pose recommended postnatally (see page 210). The hips are not lifted as high in the Pelvic Tilt, making it more suitable than the Shoulder pose for pregnancy.

The Pelvic Tilt has been recommended by several authorities on pregnancy and childbirth. In my experience, there has been no apparent discomfort or contraindications from this exercise and most women seem to enjoy the weight

being eased from their lower body. However, if you feel any discomfort in your back or fullness in the face, discontinue the exercise or do the variation below.

The Pelvic Tilt is particularly useful for relieving lower back pain. Pressure in the lower pelvic area and groin is also alleviated as the posture moves the baby a little higher into the body.

The reproductive area is toned and digestion is improved as pressure on the bowel and the organs of the digestive system is relieved when gravity is reversed. It also has a toning effect on the thighs and buttocks.

Again, due to the elevation of the pelvis, this is an ideal posture to practise regularly if you have pockets in your large intestine (diverticulitis) or haemorrhoids.

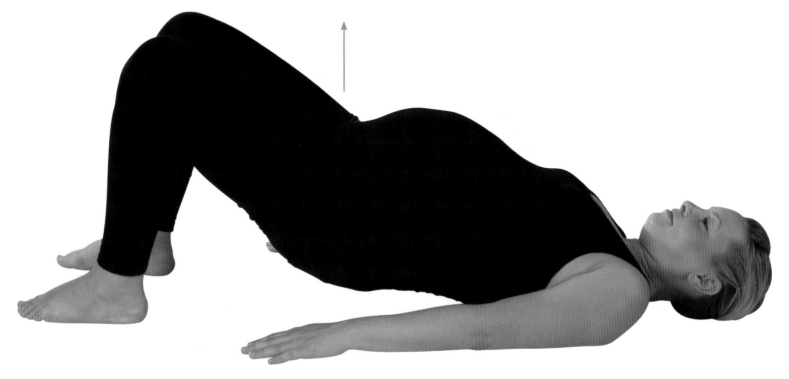

In the final posture your chin is held close to your chest, which has a normalising effect on the thyroid and parathyroid glands in your throat.

1. Lie on your back with your knees bent and your feet a little apart and flat on the floor. Place your feet as close to your buttocks as possible.
2. Breathe in and lift your hips up, keeping your head on the floor and your chin locked into the chest. Your hands can remain, palms down, on the floor or be placed under your hips for extra lift and support. Your feet stay flat on the floor.
3. Breathe out and lower your hips to the floor.
4. This can be repeated up to five times. As an alternative, you can hold the final posture for longer, while breathing and relaxing.

On completion bring your knees into your chest and gently rock from side to side, followed by coming onto your side and then resting in the Child Pose.

> **Note:** The Pelvic Tilt is sometimes recommended in cases where the baby is lying transverse or posterior, and occasionally in the breech position. Resting in this pose, and pelvic rocking on the hands and knees and avoiding leaning back while seated, can have a positive influence on moving the baby into the head-down position however, the baby might be in those positions for an internal reason and thus unable to come into the ideal birthing position. If you know your baby is in any of these positions, always seek professional advice before encouraging her to turn with these exercises. Most doctors do not like attempting to turn a breech baby due to the risks involved. If your baby is in any of these positions from about 33 weeks, it can be very helpful to spend some quiet time in meditation talking to her. If you ask your baby to move into the ideal position for birth, with the important proviso that you and your doctor are sure it is completely safe to do so, this is sometimes enough to encourage her to move into the correct position.

Variation

If the Pelvic Tilt is not comfortable, lie close to the wall on your back with your legs raised, knees slightly bent and feet flat against the wall. Position your buttocks close to the wall and lift your hips slightly to the desired height. You can also place two or three cushions under your buttocks to give you the same lift and tilt in the pelvis without the effort of holding your body up yourself. Remain in this position, relaxing into the body with your awareness on the breath. If you are carrying a lot of extra weight and there is a feeling of fullness in the face, I don't recommend this posture be practised in the last trimester.

CHAPTER 3

SQUATTING POSTURES

Because of the many benefits squatting has to offer it should always be included in pregnancy yoga classes and birth preparation. Squatting has been used for childbirth since ancient times as it is the natural, instinctive way for women to birth their babies. In many Eastern cultures and some Third World countries the squatting position is still used by many women, who often give birth with less apparent difficulty than we do in the West—their deliveries are generally shorter and need less intervention. I am not suggesting that squatting for birth automatically guarantees an easier labour. However, there are many advantages to squatting, both the full squat and modified versions. Regular practice of squatting exercises, even if you do not intend using this position for labour, is an excellent way to prepare your body for birth.

From Victorian times until the later part of the twentieth century, women in Western countries were usually required to deliver lying on their backs, a position which makes birth much more difficult.

It's like pushing uphill rather than taking into consideration anatomy, what happens during the birthing process, and the force of gravity. In Victorian times it was considered unnatural and immodest to deliver in any other way, and later was the preferred position primarily because it was easier for the medical team. Women today are more fortunate as our comfort and needs are considered very important and there is a greater understanding of the whole birthing process.

In *New Active Birth*, Janet Balaskas gives important reasons why squatting is recommended—for both mother and baby—during pregnancy and labour.

Squatting is closest to nature's laws and is known as the physiological position. A position is physiologically effective:
- *when there is no compression on the vena cava and the aorta*
- *when the pelvis becomes fully mobilised Supported squatting seems to be especially efficient at the end of the second stage when the baby is being born.*

The squatting position produces:
- *maximum pressure inside the pelvis*
- *minimum muscular effort*
- *optimal relaxation of the perineum*
- *optimal foetal oxygenation*
- *a perfect angle of descent in relation to gravity (page 14).*

Squatting is a natural position. In many countries a squatting position is used for both work and rest. Small children squat while playing and are obviously comfortably, and your child will also while playing.

The Benefits of Squatting

- The uterine and pelvic floor muscles are toned and strengthened.
- The muscles of your thighs, knees, calves and ankles are exercised and your feet are massaged in all the squatting postures. Circulation is greatly improved to your lower limbs and to your pelvic area. Stiffness is removed from your legs and hips.

- Your hips become more flexible and your lower back muscles are toned and stretched. This is particularly important during pregnancy because the lower back often develops a 'sway', sometimes causing severe pain. The squatting position reduces the curve in your back and relieves pressure on the discs of your spine as your pelvis is tilted upwards. This means that the vertebrae of your lower spine are rounded and flexed, resulting in less strain. Women suffering lower back pain, especially sciatica, in the last trimester gain excellent relief from either the full squatting postures or the modified forms recommended.

- When a woman is in labour in either the squat or a modified squatting posture, her pelvis is closer to being vertical and the child descending the birth canal can be delivered more easily. Contractions are often less intense in the squatting postures.

- The risk of uterine prolapse is lessened with regular squatting practice because the pelvic floor and inner thigh muscles are toned and strengthened. These muscles assist in supporting your uterus, bladder and other pelvic organs.

- It is recommended that people prone to constipation and haemorrhoids practise squatting as regularly as possible. Both problems are quite common during pregnancy.

- All the squatting and seated postures help to hold your spinal column straight so that your internal organs are neither cramped nor congested. This is important to remember as more efficient circulation is thus supplied to your abdominal organs.

- Squatting is very beneficial during the second stage of labour as it increases the internal diameter of the pelvis by up to 2 centimetres, or 28 per cent.

By practising the squatting postures with your partner and birth assistants during pregnancy you will become familiar with

---

Note: Before you begin the squatting exercises, practise the warming-up exercises for the feet, the hip rotations and the Butterfly to loosen your hips.

Caution: If you have varicose veins, severe pubic pain, a cervical stitch or enlarged veins in the vulva, always obtain advice from your doctor or midwife before commencing squatting exercises, which in these situations should only be done on a stool. If you have only surface veins or swollen feet, sit on a stool or practise the moving squat or postures where your body is not stationary, which will prevent any discomfort from reduced circulation. If you have a serious back injury or problems with your knees, a modified form of the full squatting position, using a stool, is always recommended.

Note: When you are in a full squatting position the space in your pelvis increases by approximately 28 per cent. If your baby is in the occiput anterior position, the ideal position for birth, and has engaged, deep squatting will encourage her to stay there, which is what you want when labour begins. If your baby is occiput posterior (facing forward with her spine against your spine, which can cause discomfort during labour) or is in the breech position you are advised not to do the full squat. Instead, do a standing squat or sit on an exercise ball so that your hips are higher than your knees, leaning your body forward. This will often encourage your baby to come into the optimum position for birth, especially if she is posterior. Standing pelvic rocking also encourages this position, which is one of the reasons it so often suggested to women during labour if a baby is posterior.

the variations you can comfortably sustain. The more practice you do the easier it will be to use them in labour. It's worth commenting that if you are planning a water birth, practising squatting in water is easier than 'on land'.

A modified 'standing squatting' position is sometimes used successfully during labour, with a birth support on either side of the woman, supporting her under the arms. Gravity is a great advantage in this position and the support of others prevents fatigue building up.

Many women find learning to squat as a adult quite challenging, but perseverance and practice are well worth the effort and initial discomfort. The modified variations are ideal alternatives that everyone can manage.

The full squatting position is practised with your feet flat on the floor, your knees wide and your spine straight. If this is too difficult a number of acceptable alternatives still provide all the benefits.

Squatting Against the Wall

You can squat with your back leaning against a wall, either on your toes or with your feet flat on the floor, and sitting on a low stool or on a stack of large books. Leaning against the wall like this is extremely comfortable and very relaxing, and greatly relieves lower back discomfort.

Squatting on a Low Stool

The stool (or pile of books) should be low enough that when you are sitting

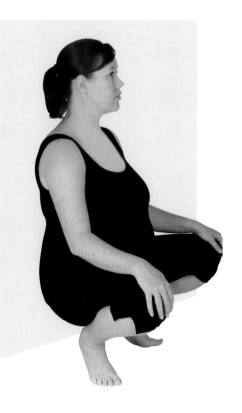

on it your knees are in line with your hips. Regularly squatting on a low stool during pregnancy is an excellent birth preparation. It can also be used as a resting position between the other squatting postures. Make yourself comfortable and lean forward resting your elbows on your knees, or place your hands on your lower legs or feet, and gently push your knees a little wider. If you prefer, join your hands in the prayer position or with fingers crossed. Gently ease the knees wider and come as far forward as you can, always in complete comfort. You might need to adjust the position of your

feet, taking them further apart or bringing them closer to the stool, for the maximum benefit. This position can be held for as long as you wish.

Squatting on a stool gives a wonderful openness to your lower back and pelvis without putting any pressure on your feet and lower legs. This position is thoroughly enjoyed by all women and highly recommended, especially if you are not able to do a full squat or you have injured your knees in the past. It is often used during labour for comfort and the benefits of gravity. Similar results can be achieved resting on a birthing chair.

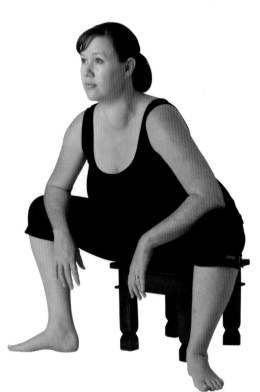

The Moving Squat

In the moving squat you transfer your weight from one foot to the other in a rocking movement from side to side. This helps your legs to become accustomed to squatting and I suggest it as a warming up exercise before practising any of the other exercises. It is recommended if you are unable to stay in the static posture for the reasons noted above, or for relief between the exercises. The rocking movement helps relieve stiffness and loosens your hips, knees and ankles. Commence this exercise from a full squatting position either on your toes or flat feet.

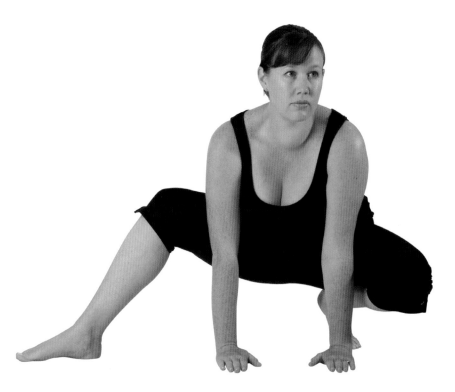

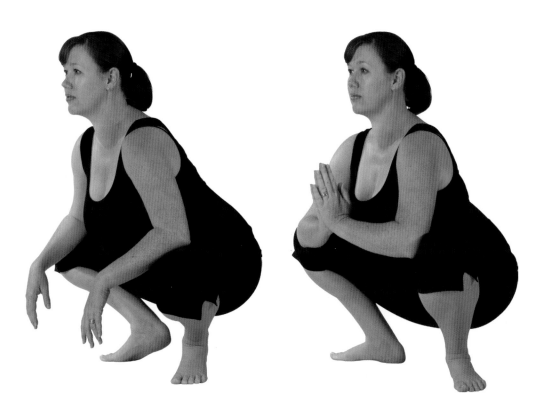

The Full Squat

1. Stand with your feet about a metre apart and turn your feet out slightly. Bend your knees and come into a full squatting posture, either on your flat feet or your toes. This can also be practised sitting on a stool or a low step. Keep your arms relaxed and rest your hands comfortably on your knees or on the floor in front of you. Have your knees wide apart and lean your body slightly forward.

2. Remain in the static posture. To ease pressure in your legs place your hands on the floor between your feet and move from one foot to the other in a rocking motion. Even if you are familiar with squatting and find it quite

comfortable, this movement will help you to relax into the posture more easily.

3. Relax into the full squatting posture and remember to breathe naturally. When you have held the squat for the desired time, return to a standing position, or place your hands behind your back and lower your buttocks to the floor, stretching your legs out in front of you.

4. From either the standing or sitting position, rotate your ankles slowly in both directions and shake your legs lightly.

Stretching and Squatting

This posture will give your hips, knees and ankles greater flexibility. Like the moving squat, it is an ideal warming-up exercise for the other squatting postures. Your legs are stretched alternately, one leg being extended to the side while the other remains bent. You will observe a deep stretch in your inner thigh area.

1. Begin in the squatting posture, with your feet flat on the floor or on your toes.

2. Place your hands on the floor between your feet. Extend your right leg to the side holding it straight, with your heel or your toes on the floor. Most of your weight will be on your left foot.

3. Change legs and take your left leg to the side. Relax into that position and repeat this up to five times each side. Do this slowly, spending some time with your leg to the side to feel the benefits of the stretch in your inner thigh, and the flexion of the hip and knee in your other leg.

The Salute Squat: *Namaskarasana*

For women who enjoy squatting, this lovely posture will supply all the benefits that squatting provides, plus a deep expansion into your groin and pelvic floor. The Salute is traditionally practised with your feet flat on the floor, but can be done on your toes, with your back against the wall or seated on a low stool.

1. Begin the Salute from the Full Squat posture. Stretch your arms forward between your knees. Join the palms of your hands together and lower your head toward your chest, being aware that your neck and shoulders remain relaxed. The outsides of your upper arms will be resting on the inside of your knees.

2. Breathe in as your hands are brought, palms together, to the centre of your chest into a prayer position. This movement will cause your elbows to gently push your knees a little wider. Straighten your back and look upwards. In this position, you will feel a deep stretch and full expansion in your hips and inner thighs. Deeper breathing becomes possible as your back is straightened and your chest is opened.

3. Breathe out as you extend your arms forward between your knees, lowering your head again.

4. Continue on with both movements, inhaling as you gently open your knees wider and look up, and exhaling as you extend your arms and lower your head.

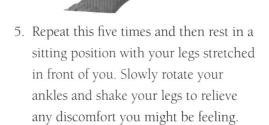

The salute squat

1. From the Full Squat position, place your hands on your lower legs or hold on to your big toe with your thumb and first finger.
2. Breathe in as you rise into a bent-over, standing position with your legs straight, holding onto your toes. If you are unable to reach your toes with your legs straight, hold onto your ankles or lower legs instead.
3. Breathe out as you bring your head in towards your legs, stretching your hamstrings. If you don't like having your head down, this stretch can be done with your head up.
4. Breathe in and look up.
5. Breathe out as you come back into the squat. The four movements of the squatting and standing

5. Repeat this five times and then rest in a sitting position with your legs stretched in front of you. Slowly rotate your ankles and shake your legs to relieve any discomfort you might be feeling.

Gas-relieving Posture: *Vayu Nishkasana*

This posture has a very beneficial effect on your whole digestive system and is useful for removing gas and discomfort from the abdominal area. It is recommended as a relief from constipation and haemorrhoids and is an excellent tonic to the nerves of your legs, arms and shoulders. With regular practice this posture will keep your body flexible and loose while supplying all the other benefits of squatting.

It is commenced from the Full Squat posture, either with your feet flat on the floor or on your toes.

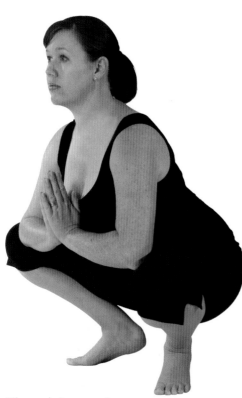

The salute squat

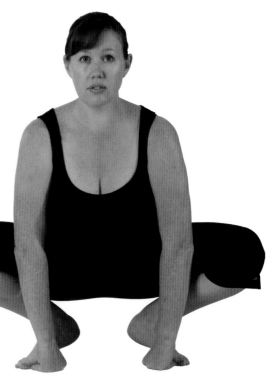

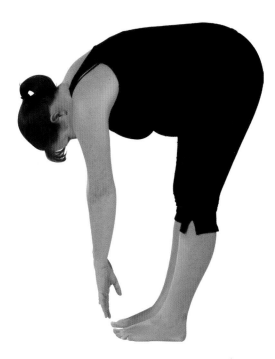

while holding the posture, or your respiration rate increases, come out of the posture immediately and rest until your breathing has returned to normal.

This is a strong posture, and with regular practice your strength and tone will quickly improve. It is an excellent posture during pregnancy as it helps create the stamina needed for labour and is one of the foremost postures to consider if you have a weak lower back.

1. Stand with your feet turned out, about a metre apart. Hold your spine straight and let your arms fall relaxed from your shoulders.

2. Breathe in to prepare and as you breathe out bend your knees and lower yourself into a deep standing squat. Make sure your pelvis is tilted slightly forward and your back is held straight. Although this makes it more strenuous it is better to hold the posture for less time and do it properly and therefore gain the real benefits. Your knees and thighs are open wide and you experience a deep inner thigh stretch. Lower yourself as deeply into the squat as you are able to in comfort and hold this final position. Keep your breathing even and your upper body relaxed. As an alternative you might like to rest your elbows on your knees, lean

exercise need to be coordinated with two full breaths.

6. The movement can be repeated five times. When you have completed the exercise, rest your legs as detailed for the other squatting postures.

The Deep Standing Squat: *Utthanasana*

Utthanasana is a very important and powerful yoga posture. It strengthens your thighs, buttocks, and importantly, the muscles of your lower back. It looks less strenuous than it is, so take care not to hold the final posture for longer than is realistic for your level of fitness and strength. If you find it especially strenuous, remain in position 2 for a shorter time until your strength improves. If you begin to feel weak and fatigued

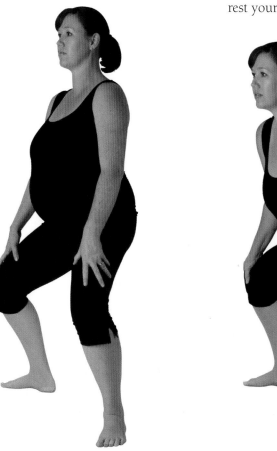

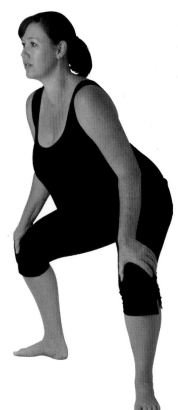

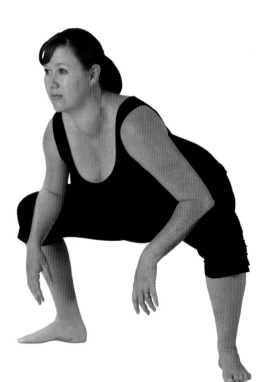

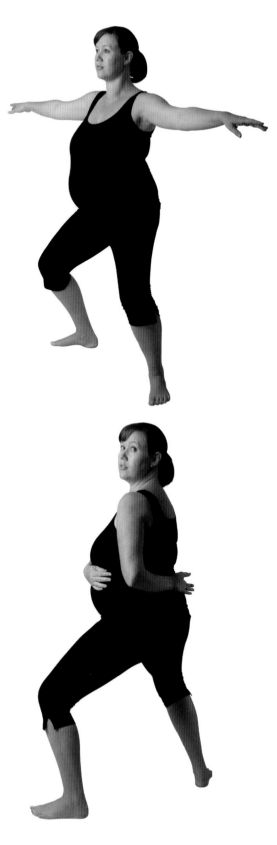

If you are quite strong and find this exercise easy, it can be held for longer while your breathing is even and relaxed. However, if you hold this posture for too long and overdo it, you will experience fatigue and might be sore for a day or two. This posture can also be practised with your lower back against the wall for extra support, and on an exercise ball.

The Deep Standing Squat with a Spinal Twist

This exercise is very relaxing for the back and is particularly good for relieving tightness and stiffness in your spine.

1. From the Deep Standing Squat position, extend your arms out to the sides.
2. Turn your body as far to the left as you can and wrap your arms around your body while looking over your left shoulder.
3. Repeat this movement on the opposite side by swinging to the right in a smooth flowing movement. Repeat this up to five times in each direction.
4. When you have completed the exercise return to the centre, lower your arms and come out of the squatting posture. When your body moves from right to left you are no longer in a static squatting position, which makes it a lot easier to do and to hold for longer.

forward slightly and ease the knees wider. This can be held for longer as is not as strenuous as the upright position, although the inner thigh stretch is greater when resting on your thighs. Try moving slowly from side to side as this lessens the demand on the body considerably.

3. Breathe in and return to the standing position. Rest and relax before repeating the posture up to three times. Each time you repeat this, try to move more deeply into it without forcing yourself into a position of discomfort or strain. When you have completed the posture move your feet closer together and shake your legs lightly.

Slow Chopping Wood

This exercise has many benefits and is usually thoroughly enjoyed, but is also the most strenuous of the yoga postures I recommend. For that reason you need to take care not to overdo it, and include it only if you are strong in the legs. It is quite easy to do and because of that there is a tendency to do more than five, which I feel is quite enough. Even if you are very strong in your legs doing more than this can result in sore thigh muscles the next day. Chopping Wood greatly improves strength in your thighs and lower back and increases tone and stamina.

1. Stand with your legs about a metre apart, your feet turned out and the hands joined in front of the body.
2. Breathe in and raise your arms above your head.
3. Breathe out through the mouth, and come into a squatting position, either onto your toes or your flat feet, and lower your arms.
4. Breathe in and return to position 2, then repeat position 3.

Repeat this three times, and no more than five times. Rest on completion and shake your legs lightly.

Note: It is easier to lean forward as you move from the standing position into the squat, but to receive the full benefits from Chopping Wood it is important to keep your pelvis tilted slightly forward and your back straight throughout and to use your thigh muscles rather than your back.

Wall Stretches

The wall stretches are alternative ways to practise the Full Squat, the Butterfly and the seated wide leg stretches. They are especially good for women who are not comfortable in the seated positions and are recommended if you have a lower back problem, or if your back problem is aggravated after practising the Wide Leg Stretch.

Even if you are flexible and enjoy the seated positions, you will feel a much deeper stretch when these three exercises are practised lying on the floor. This is because pressure is taken off your back when you are lying down and gravity is

working with you to assist the movement and 'open' more fully.

From the lying position the inner thigh stretch and the depth of tone experienced throughout the pelvic area are actually greater than from the seated positions. Most pregnant women really enjoy this way of practising and for some it becomes the preferred way of doing stretches during pregnancy and after the birth as well.

The easiest way to prepare for the wall stretches is to sit with your left hip against the wall and then lie down on your back as you swing your body around and lift

your legs up the wall. Rest your head on a cushion and place one under your hips. When your have completed these wall stretches, rest on your left side for a few minutes before coming up into a seated position, and then rest in the Child Pose.

The Wall Squat

Lie on your back with your body straight, your buttocks as close to the wall as possible and your legs straight up the wall. Separate your feet slightly as you would if you were squatting on your feet and bend your knees so that your feet are close to your buttocks, keeping your heels on the wall.

Rest your hands on the inside of your knees and gently open your knees wider, opening up through your inner thigh and pelvic region. Relax and breathe into the stretch.

> **Caution:** Please refer to Precautions (page 23) for lying on your back. Some women are not comfortable lying on their back in the last trimester, or even earlier. If this is the case discontinue the exercise immediately. If you have pubic instability or severe pain in that area please consult your midwife or a physiotherapist before practising any wide leg postures, whether from a seated position or on your back.

The Butterfly

Prepare as you did for the Wall Squat. Bring the soles of your feet together, open your knees wide and rest your hands on the inside of your knees. As you breathe out, gently ease your knees towards the wall, relaxing deeply into the position with each breath. The inner thigh stretch should feel relaxing—never over-extend into the pose. Rest from time to time and breathe into the stretch. The weight of your legs will assist with opening throughout your pelvic area and all the muscles in this part of your body will be toned and stretched.

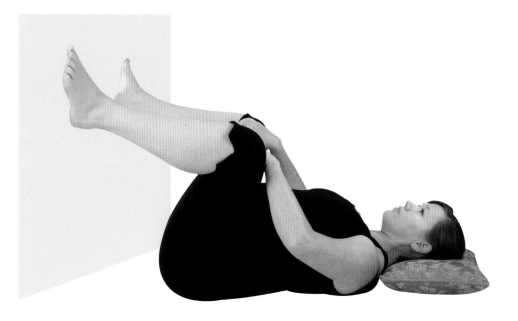

The Wide Leg Stretch

Prepare for the Wide Leg Stretch as for the Wall Squat and the Butterfly. Open your legs as wide as possible, keeping your legs straight, feeling the weight of your legs stretching your inner thighs. Relax and breathe into the stretch, holding the posture for as long as you are comfortable. The wall stretch is an ideal alternative if you are feeling short of room in your abdomen in the seated forward bend, especially in the third trimester (presuming you are comfortable resting on your back). If you are very flexible there is a risk of over-extending in this position, so rest your ankles on books or low stools so that your legs do not open as widely.

Lying with your legs straight up the wall provides great relief for tired and aching feet and fluid retention in your ankles or feet. Discomfort in the groin later in pregnancy can be relieved by placing one or two cushions under the hips in this position, or by lifting the hips slightly higher for a reduced pelvic tilt. In the elevated position the knees are slightly bent and the feet are on the wall. This is only recommended if you are relaxed and not experiencing any discomfort in your face or have shortness of breath.

CHAPTER 4

THE SPINAL TWISTS

The spinal twists are known as *matsyendrasanas* after Matsyendra, one of the founders of Hatha Yoga. This chapter includes twists practised in a seated position and lying on the floor, and range from the simplest and least demanding on your body to a slightly modified full posture that most women find very beneficial and easy to do.

No yoga program is complete without the spinal twists, which are designed to work the central network within the body—the spinal column and central nervous system. They can also be practised on their own due to the many benefits they offer. The spinal column runs the length of your body from the base of your spine, the tail bone, to the top of your spine, the atlas, at the base of your skull. It is from your central nervous system that the nerves reach all areas of your body.

Physically and emotionally there are many reasons why the spinal twists are so valuable in a pregnancy yoga program, including:

- Tension in your back—often caused by mental stress manifesting as tight muscles—is relieved with regular practice. By gently moving your body into a spinal twist, you can loosen tight muscles and soothe your nerves. You will feel more relaxed as your whole nervous system is toned and supported.
- The way we think and feel, and the way we live our lives, also has a significant bearing on the health of the nervous system. That is, our lifestyle directly affects how the body functions and the level of physical, mental and emotional health we experience in our day to day lives. The health of the nervous system, and to a lesser degree the suppleness of the spine, influences the balance and wellbeing that is experienced in the whole body.
- The spinal twists are unique as they work in a way that relaxes the physical body and calms the mind at the same time. They are really a complete yoga practice within themselves—you are in a posture that relieves tension in the physical body and works specifically on your nervous system, and has a calming restful influence on the atmosphere of your mind. The benefits are there on all levels. For these reasons they are recommended if you are under a lot of stress, or are fatigued and just can't relax enough to do some meditation.
- Your digestion is improved because the muscles and organs in your abdominal area are alternately compressed and stretched, therefore assisting optimum function.

The spinal twists will not change the way we think or our outlook on life, but they will loosen an inflexible, tense back and give us the opportunity to realise how much the way we think affects our physiology. They remind us to take more care of our physical bodies and, importantly, to be mindful of our thought processes. When they are practised regularly, you will begin to notice a greater sense of wellbeing in your body and a more relaxed, quiet awareness of your inner self. The more in tune we become with the physical body, the more likely we are to understanding our thoughts and our feelings, realising how neither one is ever really separate from the other.

The spinal twists recommended can be modified, especially in the last weeks of pregnancy, where your size might prevent you from comfortably practising some of the postures. It is important to feel as relaxed as possible when you are holding the final positions, so you can breathe and move deeply into the twist.

The spinal twists also have wonderful value after the birth. These gentle exercises very quickly help to ease the build-up of physical tension resulting from a busy day of just being a new mother, especially after a sleepless night or two. Babies are small, but if you are carrying your baby for any length of time you soon realise how even a slight weight can cause tension in your back muscles. When you are breast-feeding your posture needs to be as comfortable as possible. Full breasts are weighty, a new body experience that can mean tightness developing in neck and shoulders. A couple of spinal twists done quietly and consciously will help to release that tightness and restore energy and balance. Relaxation is very important when you are at home with your newborn. Finding the time to yourself for a little rest can be almost impossible, but you only need 10 or 15 minutes of these gentle

stretches to notice their relaxing influence. When the position is held and you are completely relaxed, and you are counting your breaths so your mind is focused and present, these postures can be likened to a meditation in movement. I often suggest to new mothers who don't have enough time for a good rest or the luxury of a massage that they hold each position for at least 15 natural breaths, with the emphasis on using the outgoing breath to relax deeply into the twist. Even the gentlest twist will bring peace of mind and softness in your body and improve your energy levels for the rest of the day.

For all the seated spinal twists, follow this procedure:

- Make sure your body is relaxed and your spine is straight before commencing the twists, using cushions to elevate the pelvis and for extra comfort and support.
- Breathe in to prepare and lift up through your spine.
- Breathe out to move into the twist.
- Breathe quietly and relax while holding the posture.
- Breathe in as you return to the front.
- Breathe out as you release the posture.

I suggest each twist be held for five breaths, but they can be held for as long as you wish, remembering to always hold each side for the same number of breaths. The longer the position is held the more benefits you will derive. Some women prefer to practice these postures with their eyes lightly closed as a way of focusing better and keeping their attention fully on the posture and the breathing. When the spinal twists are held for longer they can be done with ujjayi breathing (page 106), or breathing in through the nose and out through the mouth (page 98) to enhance the relaxation response. Done in this way they become a deeply relaxing meditation that is therapeutic and nourishing to mind and your body.

Note: When practising the seated spinal twists, try to feel as if you are twisting from the base of your spine rather than from the middle of your back. In other words, feel that you are lifting from the floor upwards. In this way your back is held straight before you begin turning and the full benefit of the posture will be experienced. Some women find it very difficult to sit with their back straight and it is quite acceptable to sit on one or two cushions for all the twists. This will serve to elevate the pelvis slightly and make it a lot easier to hold the spine upright and to twist from the base.

Seated Spinal Twists

The Easy Seated Spinal Twist:
Meru Wakrasana
This gentle exercise is an excellent way to twist the spinal column and loosen deeply throughout your back. You will feel your whole spine twisting from the base to the vertebrae of your neck.

Seated Spinal Twist with
Straight Legs
1. Sit on the floor with your legs in front of you and your spine straight.
2. Breathe in to prepare. Breathe out and turn your body to the left. Look over your left shoulder and place your left hand behind your back and your right hand on the outer part of your left thigh or left knee. Hold your spine straight and your shoulders relaxed while you relax into the twist. Hold the posture for five breaths. The arm behind your back acts as a support and also stops you from leaning back too far.
3. Breathe in as you return to the front.
4. Repeat the twist by turning to the right.

Seated Spinal Twist with
One Leg Bent

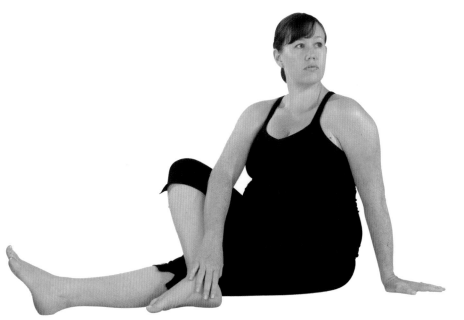

1. Sit with your spine straight and your legs in front of you. Your left leg remains straight and your right leg is bent with your right foot placed to the outside of your left knee. If this is not comfortable, place the foot to the inside of the knee.
2. Breathe in to prepare and breathe out as you turn your body to the left so you are looking over your left shoulder. Place your left hand behind your back, your right arm rests along your right inner thigh. A little pressure on the inside of your right leg will help you to move further into the twist without over-extending or forcing the posture in any way. When you are in a comfortable position, relax into the posture, holding it for five or more breaths.

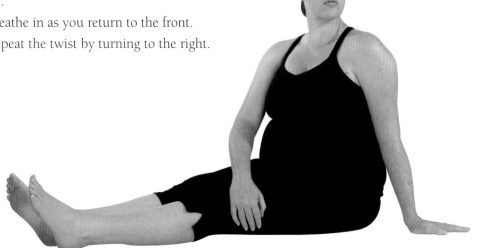

3. Breathe in as you return to the front. Change legs to repeat the twist to the right.

The following two exercises are very easy and most women enjoy doing them throughout their pregnancies, especially when some of the other twists become less comfortable.

Seated Spinal Twist with Both Legs Crossed

1. Sit in a cross-legged position.
2. Breathe in to prepare; turn to the left as you breathe out, and look over the left shoulder. The right hand is on your left knee and the left hand is behind you, supporting your back.
3. Hold this position for five breaths and relax deeply into it.
4. Breathe in as you return to the front, and then repeat this easy twist to the right.

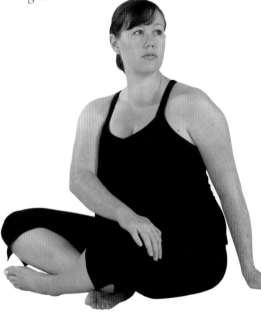

Seated Spinal Twist with Half Crossed-leg Twist

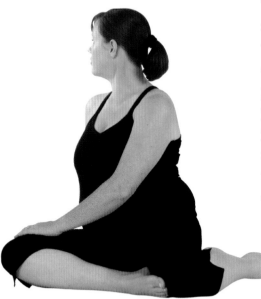

1. Cross your legs and then bend the left leg so that your left foot is facing away from the centre front and is near your left hip. The spine is straight and relaxed.
2. Turn to the right away from your legs; your right hand is behind your back giving support to your back and the left hand rests on your right knee. Hold the back as tall and straight as possible and relax into the twist for five or more breaths.
3. Return to the centre front, change legs and repeat the twist turning to your left.

Modified Full Spinal Twist: *Ardha Matsyendrasana*

This asana has been modified but retains many of its original benefits. Care needs to be taken in this posture as it is a deeper twist and stretch than the previous postures, especially through the middle of your back and your abdomen. However, if you approach both variations sensibly and in a relaxed way, it can often be practised throughout your pregnancy in complete comfort.

You need to have a reasonable level of flexibility in your hips and thighs to relax into this posture and take care not to over-extend. If you feel you are sitting a bit lop-sided and not centred, it is helpful to place a cushion first under the right hip to straighten up more, and under the left hip when the legs are reversed. This is the traditional seated position. If it can be managed in comfort you will feel balanced and very steady in the final pose.

Variation 1

1. Begin with your legs crossed.
2. Bend your right leg and place your right foot beside your left outer thigh.
3. Your left foot rests beside your right hip. Your buttocks are on the floor or on cushions, and you are sitting steady and balanced with your spine straight. This position gives a deep stretch to the right thigh and hamstring.
4. Breathe in as you turn your body to the left. Place your right arm along the inside of your right leg or, if this is not comfortable, place your right hand on your left knee to ensure that your shoulders and arms are relaxed. Your left hand is on the floor behind you. Look over your left shoulder being aware that your shoulders are completely relaxed.
5. Hold the final posture for five or more breaths.
6. Breathe in as you return to the centre front, unfolding your legs as you breathe out.
7. Repeat the twist to the other side by changing legs and turning to the right. Shake your legs a little when you have completed each side.

Variation 2

1. The legs are in the same position as for variation 1 but instead of turning away from the legs, this time you will be turning your body in the opposite direction. This is not suitable for everyone but it is worth recommending because many women enjoy this twist to full-term pregnancy.

   Turn your body to the left, place your left hand on the floor behind your back and rest your right hand either on your right knee or your left foot. This variation prevents tightness in your upper body and arms. You will feel a gentle twist in your abdominal area as well as in the middle of your back.
2. Breathe out as you turn your head and look over your left shoulder. Breathe and relax into this lovely posture.
3. Breathe in as you turn your body to the front. Breathe out as you unfold your legs. Shake your legs lightly.
4. Repeat the twist to the other side.

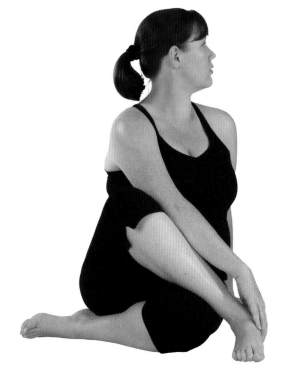

Half spinal twist

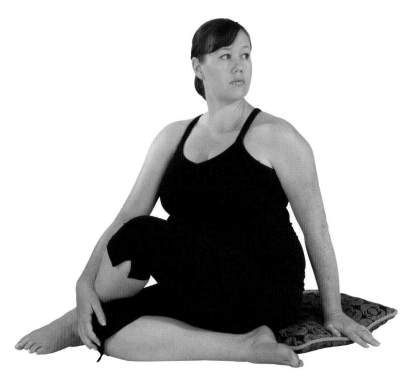

Full spinal twist

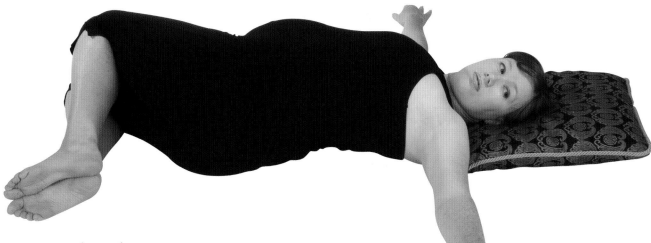

It is important not to twist beyond your level of flexibility. Practise these twists as often as possible and you will soon notice an improvement. Be aware not to hold tension in your shoulders or your back when you are in the full posture. As you relax and breathe into all these positions, imagine tightness and discomfort being dissolved and removed from your whole back and spinal column.

Spinal Twists on Your Back

Spinal Twist with Both Legs Bent: *Supta Udarakarshanasana*

This exercise is good for relieving tightness in your lower back and hips and is the easier of the two.

1. Lie on your back with both legs bent, your feet flat on the floor about hip-distance apart and as close to your buttocks as possible. Place a flat cushion under your head for comfort. Spread your arms along the floor at shoulder height with your palms facing down.

2. Breathe in to prepare. Breathe out as you lower your knees to the right and turn your head to face the left. Hold this for 3 breaths and relax into the twist. Let your knees drop as close to the floor as possible without your left shoulder lifting from the floor. If you are experiencing any discomfort in your lower back or hips, or are feeling too much stretch in your abdomen, lift your knees away from the floor slightly and rest them on a cushion.

3. Breathe in as you bring your knees to the upright position again.

4. Breathe out as you lower your knees to the left and turn your head to the right. Again, hold the posture as you breathe and relax deeply into your back muscles and spinal column. This can be repeated up to five times each side.

5. As an alternative, repeat the exercise moving from side to side with each breath. Breathe in with your knees in the upright position, breathe out as you take them to the right and your head to the left, breathe in as you bring them to the upright position again and breathe out as you take them to the left, and your head to the right. This can be repeated as many times as you wish and is a lovely way to relieve lower back tension and discomfort.

Note: Some women are not comfortable lying on their backs later in pregnancy. If there is any discomfort or nausea, please practise the seated postures instead. Refer to how best to move from a seated position to lying on the floor (page 23).

On completion of either variation hug your knees into your body and rock from side to side to gently massage your lower back.

Spinal Twist with One Leg Bent and One Leg Straight: *Shava Udarakarshanasana*

I often recommend this exercise if there is tension in the back or if stiffness in the spine is causing a problem, repeating it morning and night. It is very interesting to notice just how much tightness can build up in the body in the course of a day. This is one of the best ways to practise the spinal twists as you don't have to be concerned whether your spine is straight.

1. Begin by lying on your back with your spine straight, with a low cushion under your head if this is more comfortable.
2. The left leg is straight. Bend your right leg and place your right foot either behind your left knee or outside it. Choose for comfort as the foot position will not alter the effects of the posture.

3. Roll over slightly onto your left hip so that your right knee comes as close to the floor as possible without over-extending. It is important not to roll over to the point where the posture is no longer comfortable. A pillow or some cushions can be placed under the knee for comfort. Rest your left hand on your right knee. This will put weight on your knee and help to keep your body in the twisted position.
4. Extend your right arm along the floor at shoulder level with your palm facing up. Turn your head to look at your hand and place your arm where you can easily see your hand without straining your eyes or neck. If your right shoulder lifts off the floor, you have twisted too far to the left, so roll out of the twist slightly to a point where your shoulder stays on the floor. If you are holding any tension in your

right hip and lower back, roll out of the twist a little until you can relax completely.
6. Hold the final twist for five breaths or longer. The idea is to be as comfortable as if you were lying with your body straight in the relaxation posture.
7. Straighten your body to come out of the twist then repeat the posture to the other side, reversing all the movements.

Some women find this twist less comfortable as they progress through their pregnancies; if this happens to you, practise the previous twist with both legs bent.

CHAPTER 5

THE POSE OF THE CHILD

Sishuasana, the Pose of the Child (referred to throughout as the Child Pose), is such an important posture for pregnancy, birth and after the birth that it is worthy of a chapter of its own. Modified to suit individual needs, it can be enjoyed by all pregnant women. It is always a favourite relaxation position in my birth preparation classes, and after the birth too. It is a pose of deep relaxation for the mind and has many other benefits for the physical body. This posture is so named because it resembles the foetal position. It is not uncommon to see small children sleeping this way, totally relaxed and at peace.

The Child Pose is the posture of choice to relieve all forms of mental and emotional stress. A short time spent in this posture will bring quietness to your mind, a slowing down of thoughts, quieter breathing and deep relaxation in your whole body. It is a wonderful posture to do if your mind is overloaded with unwanted thoughts or it seems impossible to rest. With your head placed either on the floor or on your folded hands, the increased blood flow to your head gently stimulates the relaxation centres of your brain. This exercise is a valuable life skill and I am sure you will still be using it long after the birth of your baby.

Some people relax more in the Child Pose than any other position because it creates a feeling of safety and nurturing. You will notice your breathing slowing down the longer you hold the posture and a deep sense of peace coming over you. Many women use this position at home for relaxation and especially to relieve back problems; some even like to sleep like this.

It also greatly relieves the more common discomforts of pregnancy, especially lower back pain, sciatica and pelvic discomfort, and is often used during labour for this purpose. The slightly elevated variation is often recommended to help turn a baby who is in the posterior position during pregnancy, and during labour will relieve much of the discomfort associated with a baby being in that position. If you are in an all fours position during labour, relaxing into the Child Pose or a modified variation between contractions is very restful and also beneficial to the mood of your labour.

It is an ideal position for your partner or birth support to give you a lovely aromatherapy massage during pregnancy and especially during labour.

In these variations your knees are further apart than in the classic pose to accommodate the increasing size of your abdomen. You will notice a deep stretch to your inner thigh area and enjoy a lovely openness into the lower back. The Child Pose is not meant to be an intense stretch and should always be comfortable, relaxing and rewarding. Because of the many benefits I also teach the alternatives in my regular yoga classes.

> **Note:** There are no contra-indications for people with high blood pressure, even though your head is down and below your heart.

Seven Variations of the Child Pose

For all seven variations begin by sitting in the Thunderbolt posture (page 38). Have your knees as wide as is comfortable and your toes together. Lean forward to find the best position. Close your eyes lightly and breathe naturally and enjoy this lovely posture. Relax completely in your mind and your body.

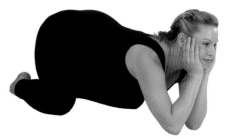

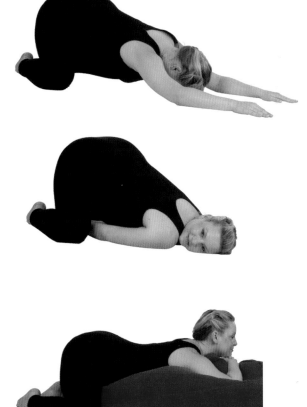

1. The head resting in the hands looking ahead. This is good if you don't like having your head down or if you are using the position to watch television, etc.

2. The head resting on folded hands. The more forward position here gives a deeper stretch through your back and is more relaxing for your mind than the previous one, because your head is lower.

3. The head on the floor with the arms beside the legs.

4. The head on the floor with the arms stretched out in front of you. Another much-liked variation—when your arms are stretched out in front you will feel a lovely stretch along the length of your back.

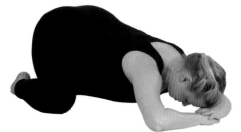

5. The head on the floor with the hands between the legs touching the toes. Your baby will probably sleep like this. Some women really enjoy this position, as it makes them feel cosy and safe.

6. Resting over a bean bag. This is an ideal option if you are intending to spend a lot of time in the Child Pose.

If you are labouring on the hands and knees you might that find resting over the bean bag between contractions is a very comfortable way to rest and relax. You can lean slightly forward so that your hips are higher than in the previous positions and for more comfort place some cushions at the back of your thighs as well.

7. Any of the above with the hips raised slightly. When the hips are raised any pressure or discomfort in the pelvis and groin will be greatly alleviated as the weight is taken away from those areas. This elevated position provides considerably more relief from lower back pain or pelvic pain than the other positions I have recommended.

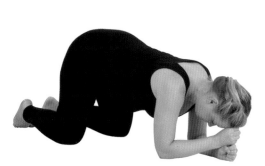

For greater comfort and support all of these can be done sitting on one or two cushions. If you have knee problems, varicose veins or swollen feet always add extra cushions, use the elevated position or use the bean bag.

CHAPTER 6

STANDING POSTURES AND EXERCISES

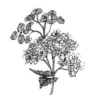

The standing yoga postures in this chapter are ideal to practise throughout your pregnancy and are mostly easy to do. They give a lovely stretch while toning your whole body, and many of them increase stamina and flexibility. Some are quite strenuous and more demanding on the body, so care needs to be taken not to overdo them—they are not recommended if you are fatigued or low in energy. The exercises and postures in this chapter can be done on their own, or in combination with those from other chapters.

For all postures that commence from a standing position, always be aware that your shoulders are relaxed and that you are not standing with an exaggerated arch in your lower back. This is important because as your pregnancy progresses you might be more inclined to have extra curve in your back which leads to discomfort and backache. To overcome this and ensure correct posture tilt your hips and pelvis slightly forward.

Hand and Finger Exercises
These exercises help maintain flexibility in your wrists, hands and fingers, and improve circulation in your lower arms. They are especially useful if your hands are inclined to swell in hot weather, if you spend a lot of time on the computer, and especially if you develop carpal tunnel syndrome during your pregnancy. They can be practised either sitting in a chair with your back straight, or standing with your feet a little apart.

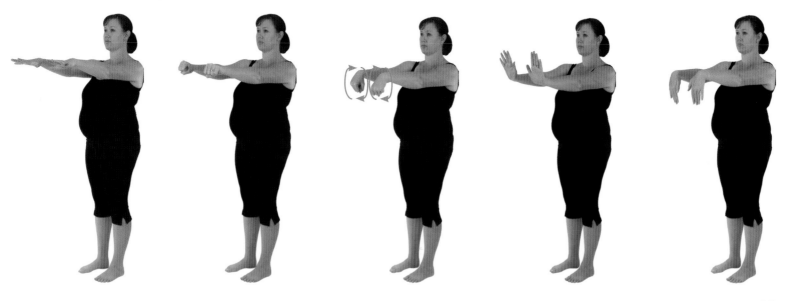

1. Stretch your arms out in front of you at shoulder height. Spread your fingers wide, then squeeze your hands into tight fists. Repeat this up to five times and hold each movement to receive the most benefit. Lightly shake your hands when you have completed the exercise.

2. Clench your fists and very slowly rotate them clockwise five times and then anticlockwise five times. As you do this, be aware of the deep stretch throughout your wrists and arms.

3. Stretch your arms out in front of you at shoulder height with palms facing down. Flex your hands upwards so that the palms are facing away from you and your fingers are pointing up. Reverse the movement and point your fingers down towards the floor. Repeat this five times, then lightly shake your hands.

Head and Neck Exercises: *Gardhanasanas*

This is an important group of exercises that helps to reduce tension in your neck and shoulders. Your neck plays a vital role in overall health because nerves from various parts of your body pass through it to your brain. If you are suffering from headaches and neck tension, regular

Caution: A full head rotation is never recommended, especially if you have a weak or injured neck.

practice of these exercises and the following shoulder exercises will provide you with welcome relief, and at the very least, will prevent the problem becoming worse.

These three exercises are best done slowly, with your upper body relaxed and your back straight. They can be done standing, sitting in a chair or sitting on the floor, with awareness that your back is straight and relaxed.

1. Lower your head towards your left shoulder, being careful not to lift your shoulder or become tense. Remember to keep the muscles in your neck and shoulders relaxed. Do not force your head over towards your shoulder

in any way and only go as far as is comfortable. Hold this position for four or five breaths, return to the vertical, and repeat it to the right. This whole exercise can be repeated as many times as desired. The weight of your head will gently stretch the muscles at the side of your neck so there is no need to force the position. It is worth doing this exercise in front of a mirror to make sure your body is not leaning as you move your head.

2. Turn your head as far to the right as possible, holding it for a short time before centring and turning to the left. Repeat this five times each side, keeping your neck and shoulders relaxed at all times.

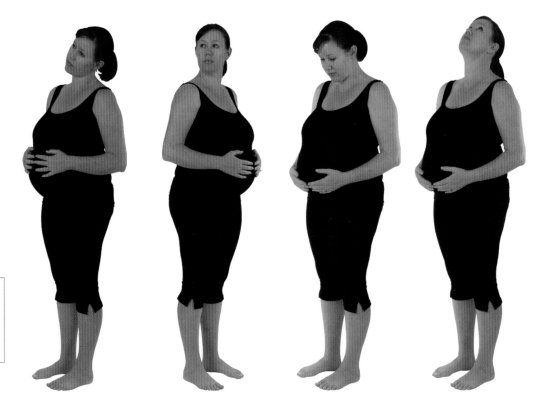

3. Drop your head down so that your chin is close to your chest. Be aware of feeling a deep stretch through the muscles of your upper back, shoulders and the central muscles of your neck. Your head can also be taken back, but I do not recommend this if you have had a neck injury. If you are able to take your head back comfortably, slowly open and close your mouth so as to stretch the muscles of your throat. Again, the weight of your head will automatically cause your neck muscles to be stretched.

Shoulder Exercise: *Shandhachakra*

This exercise helps to free tension from your shoulders and upper body. It will assist in opening up your chest for more efficient breathing and also help prevent incorrect posture and round shoulders.

1. Stand with your feet slightly apart and your body relaxed.
2. Place your fingertips on your shoulders and make slow, large circles with your elbows so that your shoulders are rotating deeply in their sockets. Repeat this five times forwards and then five times backwards. When your elbows are forward, the stretch will be felt across your upper back and shoulders helping to relieve any tension in these parts of your body. As your elbows are back, the stretch is felt in your chest. Although this is a simple exercise, the way your back and shoulders will feel

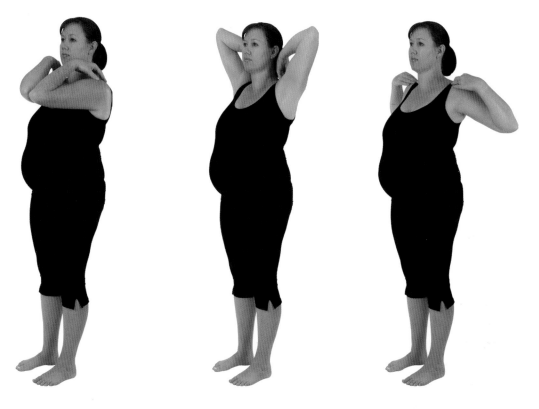

afterwards is evidence enough of its benefits. Lightly shake your arms and loosen your shoulders after the exercise is completed.

Chest Expansion with Deep Breathing: *Hasta Utthanasana*

There are many benefits from practising *hasta utthanasana*, particularly for your chest, arms, shoulders and upper back. When your arms are behind you, your chest is open and expands fully, which assists in efficient deep breathing. Many people hold tension in the muscles of their chest, upper back and shoulders and this exercise works on easing that tightness. It also helps to reduce tension in the muscles of your neck, especially when done with

the head and neck exercises.

When this exercise is practised regularly, all the muscles of your upper body are massaged. Your arms are stretched and toned and your shoulder joints are kept flexible, mobile and free. Circulation is improved to your lungs and upper body. This is also a very appropriate exercise for people who have round shoulders, poor posture and inefficient breathing. People with respiratory disorders such as asthma or emphysema are encouraged to practise this exercise and the previous one as often as possible, especially before the breathing exercises. The Chest Expansion is one of the few postures to work deeply and thoroughly into your upper body. I recommend practising it in the morning to loosen your body and at the end of the day to relieve any tightness that may have built up.

1. Stand with your body straight and your shoulders and arms relaxed. Place your right hand in front of your left hand. Keep your arms straight and relaxed.

2. Breathe in as you raise your arms up in front of your body, finishing the inhalation when your arms are above your head.

3. Breathe out as you take your arms back as far as possible while expanding your chest. When your chest is fully opened you will feel your shoulder blades come closer together and the muscles of your upper back squeeze gently.

Repeat this sequence five or more times, being aware to inhale and exhale deeply with your arm movements. The sequence also be repeated more slowly, taking two or three breaths to complete the exercise and holding your arms above your head for longer, to enjoy a full stretch in the upper body.

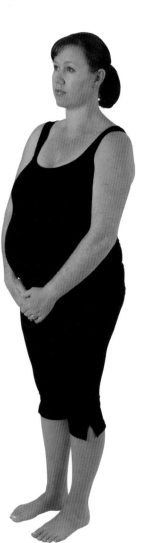

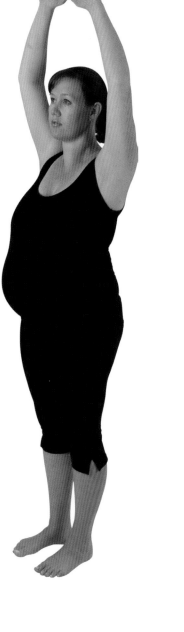

The Heavenly Stretch: *Tadasana*

This lovely posture stretches deeply yet gently throughout your spinal column, giving you the feeling of being tall, balanced and centred. The Heavenly Stretch helps remove congestion in the nerves and muscles of your spine, giving health and suppleness throughout your back. Your feet and lower leg muscles are strengthened and your feet receive extra benefits from balancing on your toes. It is helpful to focus on a stationary object before commencing the practice because it requires balance and steadiness to stretch while on your toes. If you are unsteady on your toes it is quite acceptable to practise this posture standing on flat feet.

The Heavenly Stretch is an excellent posture if constipation is a problem because it tones your abdominal muscles and intestinal area. To help overcome mild constipation, before breakfast drink two or three glasses of warm water with a squeeze of lemon juice and then practise the Heavenly Stretch, a side bend (page 71) and some spinal twists (page 56). This will often stimulate your liver and intestines enough to promote a normal bowel movement. It is a wonderfully natural way to restore normal bowel function without the use of laxatives.

1. Stand with your feet together or a little apart. Join your hands together in front of you with your palms facing upwards and your shoulders relaxed.

2. Breathe in as you raise your arms above your head, rising up onto your toes and balancing, with your palms facing the ceiling. Keep your shoulders relaxed and hold your breath briefly while you balance on your toes. It is not recommended that you hold your breath for lengthy periods during pregnancy, but a short pause is quite acceptable and will not cause you any distress.

3. Breathe out as you lower your arms and heels to the floor and return to the standing position. Repeat this five times.

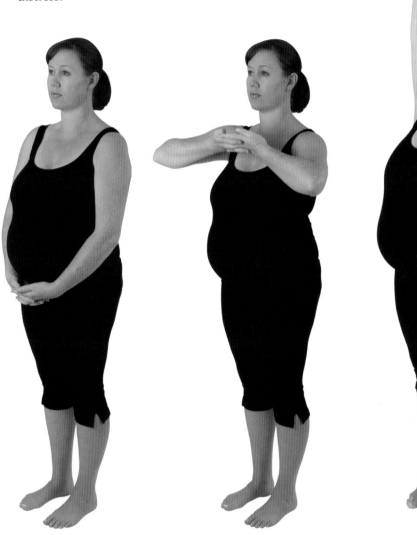

Pelvic Rocking

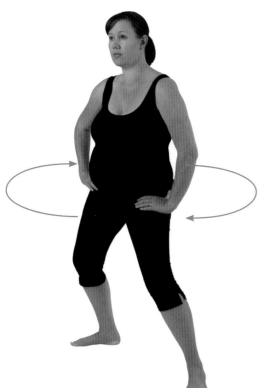

Although Pelvic Rocking is not a traditional yoga exercise, it offers many important benefits during pregnancy, and is fun to do. Stand with your feet hip-distance apart and bend your knees slightly. Make big slow circles with your hips—as a guide, rotate your hips five times clockwise and then five times anti-clockwise. It has a lovely massaging effect on your hips and pelvic area and helps to free tension from the lower body. It is often recommended during labour as it is very relaxing to the pelvic area and gravity encourages the baby to descend into the birth canal in this position. Pelvic Rocking (page 37) can also be practised on your hands and knees.

Waist Rotation and Spinal Twist:
Kati Chakrasana

When this exercise is practised regularly your spine is loosened in preparation for all other forward bending, sideways bending and spinal twist postures. It also helps relieve stiffness and tightness in the shoulders and back, and tones the waist area. This exercise is ideal to do before the spinal twists, both those done in a seated position and those lying on your back (pages 58-62).

1. Stand with your feet about hip-distance apart. Breathe in while raising your arms to the sides at shoulder height.

2. Breathe out and turn to the left, wrapping your arms around your body and looking over your left shoulder; hold this for three or four natural breaths.

3. Breathe in and return to the centre front with your arms extended to the side.

4. Breathe out and turn your body to the right, looking over your right shoulder, again holding it while you relax and breathe.

Repeat this sequence up three times each side, then repeat five times, moving more quickly from one side to the other.

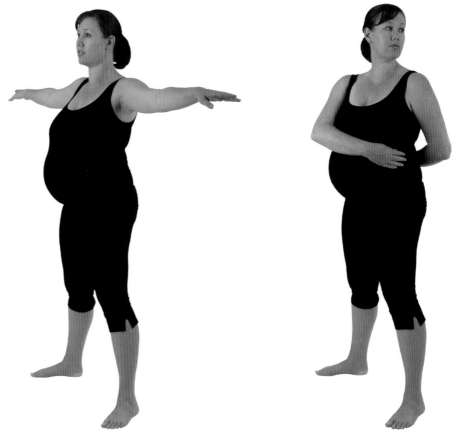

The Triangle Side Bend:
Trikonasana

Trikonasana, the full side bending posture, is a significant practice with many benefits. It is completely safe to practise during pregnancy but if you find the full side bend uncomfortable, particularly in the last few weeks, it can be modified. Some people are very supple in all the sideways bending positions but others will find the spinal twists or the forward bends easier to do. The important point to remember is how the posture is practised—with the emphasis on full body, mind and breath awareness rather than how far you have extended into the side bend.

The Triangle Side Bend is quite a dynamic posture and you need to be quite precise in the way your body is positioned to achieve all the benefits it offers. The ideal position of the final posture is to have your right ear, right shoulder and right knee in line, so that your left shoulder does not come forward. When it is practised in this way, the degree of sideways movement will be less but the final posture will be more exact.

This is a most enjoyable stretch to practise during pregnancy. The sides of your body receive either a full stretch or a deep squeeze depending on the way you are bending. As your body is taken to the right, your liver and the right side of your bowel are massaged, which assists in establishing optimum function while the left side is extended and stretched.

This is important if there are problems with a sluggish liver, minor digestive disorders or constipation. Then, as your body leans to the left, your spleen and pancreas benefit and the left side of your bowel is massaged. Bending either way gives a lovely stretch through the side of your body and into your hip. Your spinal column is stretched sideways, increasing flexibility, and your lower back, hip and inner thigh muscles are stretched.

Trikonasana is a good example of a 'passive yet dynamic' yoga posture, in that it is enjoyable and gentle, but at the same time benefits many parts of your body. I recommend this posture be included in all your yoga programs.

1. Stand with your feet about hip-distance apart, or a little wider if it's comfortable. Your left foot is facing to the front and your right foot turned out to the right. Keep your hips and shoulders in line and square to the front.

2. Breathe in and raise your arms to the sides at shoulder height, keeping your shoulders relaxed. Feel the energy flowing from your shoulders to your fingertips as you stretch your arms.

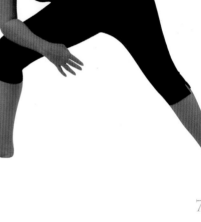

3. Breathe out and bend your body to the right. Rest your right hand on your right leg. Raise your left arm to a vertical position and gaze at your left thumb. At this point, if you feel dizzy looking up or have neck problems, look straight ahead instead, or at the floor. An alternative arm position is to extend your arm along the side of your face where you will feel a deeper stretch through the side of your body. If this is too strong continue with the previous option. Adjust the position where your hand rests on your leg to modify the depth of the side bend and only bend as far as your level of flexibility allows, never straining. Remain relaxed while holding the final posture and breathe quietly for five breaths.

4. Breathe in as you return to the standing position, then lower your arms while breathing out. Repeat the side bend to the left, reversing all the procedures.

Variation

The Triangle Side Bend can also be practised from a kneeling position, which some women prefer. The benefits are the same. Resting on your knees, extend your right leg to the side with the foot or your heel on the floor. The left knee and hip are in line so you are not over-extending. Proceed as for the standing side bend—rest your right hand on your right leg and have your left arm either straight up or extended along the side of your face for the full stretch. Look straight ahead and be aware not to over-stretch in the final position. Repeat this with the left leg to the side and bend to the left.

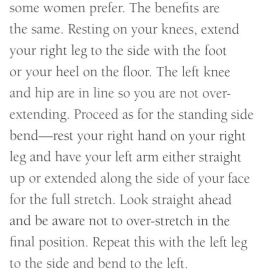

Note: To reduce the degree of the side bend, when bending to the right you might prefer to place a low stool beside your right foot and rest your hand on that rather than having your hand on your leg. It is also acceptable to have your knee bent instead of straight, especially if you are finding the inner thigh stretch too strong or have knee problems. For example, when you are bending to the right, your right knee can be slightly bent and your right hand or elbow can rest on your knee. The benefits to the side of your body are exactly the same.

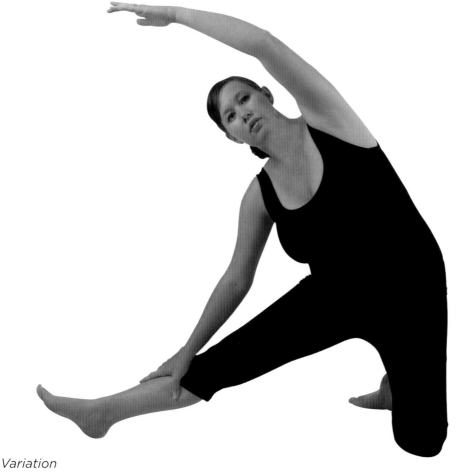

Variation

The Hero: *Virasana*

The Hero is another of the triangle postures, and like *trikonasana* is a passive but dynamic exercise. It looks fairly simple and straightforward but care needs to be taken not to hold the final posture for too long, as fatigue will result from overexertion. These strong, static yoga postures are beneficial for building strength, tenacity and endurance in the physical body. They influence mental and emotional stamina and help to develop the much sought after inner strength so important during labour.

Specifically, the Hero will strengthen your thigh, inner thigh and calf muscles while bringing tone to your whole body. Because your arms are held up and stretched they will become stronger the more the posture is practised. The Hero will also give you a feeling of balance and steadiness.

1. Stand with your feet at least a metre apart. Turn your right foot to the right and your left foot to the front. Face your body square to the front and turn your head to the right. For maximum benefits, make sure your feet are wide enough apart for you to move deeply into the posture.

2. Inhale as you raise your arms to the sides, looking out along your right arm, and then exhale while bending your right leg, keeping your lower leg vertical from ankle to knee. You will feel a deep stretch up the inside of your left leg and strength in your right thigh. Relax your shoulders and feel a strong stretch along your arms through to your fingertips. Hold this posture for five breaths, or if you are finding it quite easy hold it for longer.

3. Inhale as you straighten your right leg, then exhale as you lower your arms.

4. Repeat to your left, reversing the directions.

5. Shake your legs lightly when you have completed the posture.

If you are quite fit and find this easy to do, you might like to widen your legs and move more deeply into the final position while maintaining the correct body position.

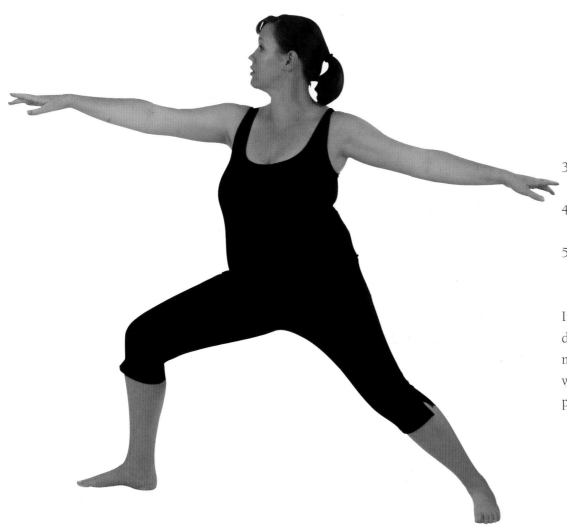

Variation: The Hero in Pairs

The Hero can also be done working with a partner. This often makes it easier and means you are able to move into the pose more deeply. Stand with your feet apart as for the Hero, with the outsides of your feet together (her right foot next to your left foot). Join hands. Bend your right knee so you are moving to the right, she does the opposite and moves to the left. The arms are straight and you lean off each other in a balanced way without either of you pulling the other off centre. Don't over-extend but enjoy the support from your partner. Relax, then repeat, reversing the directions.

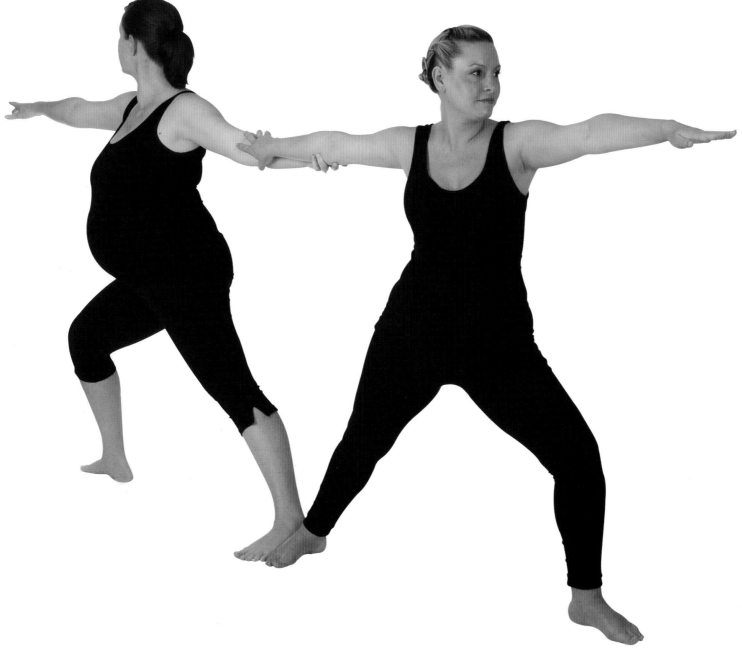

CHAPTER 6: Standing postures and exercises

The Warrior: *Virabhadrasana*

The Warrior is another of the triangle postures. It benefits your legs and increases your strength and endurance. I have modified the traditional posture slightly because I feel the full posture—where your arms are up above your head—is generally too strenuous for pregnant women.

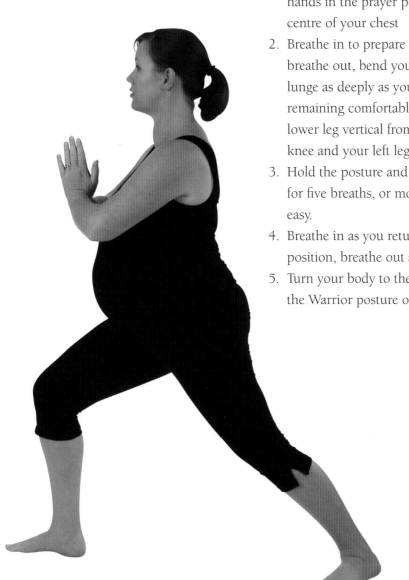

1. Stand with your feet wide apart and your toes facing forward. Turn your body to the right. Your right foot faces in the same direction as the front of your body and your left foot is turned slightly inwards. Make sure you feel steady and balanced in this position and feel a stretch in your left calf muscle and your ankle. Join your hands in the prayer position at the centre of your chest

2. Breathe in to prepare then, as you breathe out, bend your right leg and lunge as deeply as you can while remaining comfortable. Keep your right lower leg vertical from the ankle to the knee and your left leg straight.

3. Hold the posture and breathe quietly for five breaths, or more if you find it easy.

4. Breathe in as you return to the standing position, breathe out and relax.

5. Turn your body to the left and repeat the Warrior posture on that side.

The Standing Head-down Postures

There are many benefits from the head-down postures.

- Sinus congestion can be relieved and is often completely removed because your nose and nasal passages receive extra blood flow.

- Often these postures will help to alleviate mild headaches, as the weight of your head will stretch your neck muscles, relieving tension and tightness in this area.

- Circulation to your head and especially your brain is improved. Memory and concentration are also enhanced, and mental fatigue is removed. If these postures are practised around 2 to 3 p.m. (when gravity is at its greatest), you will notice an increased clarity and general alertness for the remainder of the day.

Caution: If you have a history of high or low blood pressure, or tend to become dizzy and light-headed, ask your doctor for advice before doing any of the head-down postures, and if you are attending a class inform your teacher so she is aware of your situation. If you wish to proceed always return to a standing position very, very gradually, taking two or three breaths as you do so

- Blood flow to the pituitary gland—the master gland of the endocrine system—is improved, helping to enhance the function of the whole hormonal system.
- The nervous system is balanced when the head is down, which encourages the relief of mental and emotional stress, and allows greater harmony to be experienced throughout the body and the mind. You will also appreciate an improvement in physical wellbeing.
- Your hair and scalp are kept healthy due to the increased blood supply to your head, and problems such as dandruff can sometimes be rectified with regular practice.
- As the blood flow to your face is greatly improved, your eyes and the muscles around your eyes will benefit. The head-down postures ease facial tension and are said to help prevent wrinkles.

The Pose of Two Angles:
Dwi Konasana

This is an excellent posture for removing tightness from your shoulders and upper back. When the muscles between your shoulder blades become sore due to stress or poor posture, extending your arms up behind your back is an effective way of loosening them. Dwi konasana is also one of the few exercises to work effectively into the muscles of your upper arms. When people first attempt this posture it is quite common for their arms not to extend very far away from their back. With practice,

however, your arms, shoulders and chest will free up enough for you to notice a considerable difference in extension. This exercise expands your chest muscles in a similar way to *hasta uttanasana* (page 67), and this helps establish more efficient breathing.

1. Stand with your feet facing the front about hip-distance apart. Join your hands together behind your back and relax your shoulders.
2. Breathe in to prepare and as you breathe out bend your body forward. The top of your head should be facing the floor. Extend your arms away from your body as far as is comfortable.

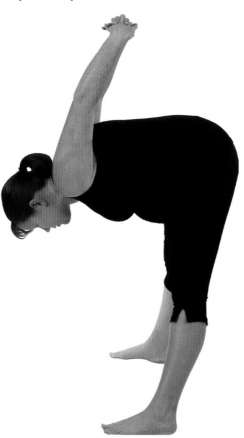

Hold this posture as you breathe in a relaxed and natural manner.

3. Breathe in as you return very slowly to a standing position. This exercise can be repeated up to three times. It can also be included in the standing Wide-A Leg Stretch below as an alternative to resting your hands on the floor, a stool or your lower legs.

Wide-A Leg Stretch:
Prasavita Padottanasana

The Wide-A Leg Stretch is a strong posture which gives a deep stretch to your inner thigh muscles and throughout your back. Before practising this stretch, check whether you are able to comfortably and easily reach the floor with your hands, without bending your knees or straining your inner thigh muscles or back.

When you first attempt this posture, begin by resting your hands on a low step, a stool or the seat of a chair, rather than trying to reach the floor. Later, you can gradually ease into the full posture without the risk of straining your body. With practice, your inner thigh and back muscles will become more flexible and you might be able to reach closer to the floor with your hands. It can also be done leaning on your kitchen table or with your hands against the wall.

Your inner thigh muscles and the muscles and ligaments of your pelvic floor are toned deeply by this wide leg stretch, thus preparing these muscles for childbirth. Your back and neck muscles

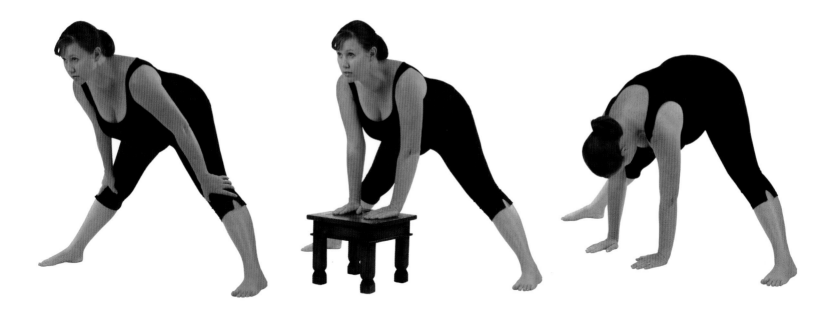

receive a good stretch and your lower back is opened and lightly stretched also. Most pregnant women really enjoy this posture for the lovely stretch it gives, while the head down position is always relaxing for the mind. This stretch is especially helpful if sciatica is a problem or where there is tightness in the shoulders and neck.

This posture is also recommended for later in pregnancy, when many women can experience considerable strain in the groin area due to the extra weight. Those who suffer diastasis symphysis pubis (DSP), a very painful problem in the pubic bones, or are carrying their baby low in the pelvis, also benefit. Leaning forward also relieves discomfort in the abdomen if the baby is still quite high late in pregnancy and you feel as if there's no room left, as this posture gives a feeling that the weight is moved away from these areas.

1. Begin by standing with your feet about a metre apart and slowly separate your legs to a distance that is comfortable for you, with your feet facing the front. If you feel the stretch is too tight, bring the feet closer together until your flexibility improves. When your legs are in position, lower your hands to a stool, or to rest on your legs, and drop your head down so that the top of your head is facing the floor. If you are able to, lower your hands to the floor. In the final position remember to feel only a light stretch in the inner thigh, never straining. You must always take full responsibility for how you are feeling in a posture and only work within your own level of flexibility and in complete comfort.

2. Hold the final posture for up to nine breaths. You will notice that the longer you remain in this posture the more relaxed your back and inner thigh muscles become as you breathe and move more completely into the stretch, and your mind will gradually become quiet and very calm.

3. When you are ready to come out of the pose bring your feet closer together and stand up very slowly while breathing in, taking at least two breaths to return to the standing position. Shake your legs lightly when the posture is completed.

If you have high or low blood pressure this can still be done for the benefits it gives to the legs and lower body. Rest your hands on a stool or on your legs and look straight ahead instead of having your head down.

The Mountain: *Parvatasana*

This wonderful posture has been called both the Mountain and the Downward Dog (*adho mukha svanasana*) in traditional yoga texts and both names describe it well. This posture resembles a dog stretching and pulling its body strongly towards its back legs. It also looks like a mountain peak, your buttocks and lower back being the summit, your arms and head resembling one side of the mountain and your legs and feet the other side.

It is probably one of the best postures for extending your hamstrings and thigh muscles and for deeply stretching your back. However, because it can be quite an intense posture and it is important to ease slowly into the full stretch and only have your heels as close to the floor as you can manage in comfort. Some people can rest their heels on the floor quite easily, others cannot, and it should be remembered this is not the main emphasis of the posture.

On first attempting this posture many people comment on how strong the stretch is and realise how tight their hamstrings and thigh muscles really are. Do not be discouraged, because with time this can become an enjoyable posture and the benefits definitely outweigh any beginner's discomfort. The majority of women enjoy this posture during pregnancy but some find it too challenging. If you find it's not for you, practise one of the other inverted postures instead or the alternative position below.

The Mountain's benefits include all those listed for the inverted postures where your head is lower than your heart. Other benefits include:

- Tightness and tension are released from your hamstrings, thigh and calf muscles, and your ankles become more flexible.
- Your spinal column is stretched and your spinal nerves are toned which has a nourishing and rejuvenating effect on your whole body.
- The muscles of your back are extended fully, keeping your back flexible and strong.
- Tired and aching legs are relieved, muscle cramps are often removed and circulation to your legs is generally improved.
- It is one of the postures recommended for relieving backache or sciatic pain, both common problems during pregnancy.
- Circulation to your arms and hands is increased. The Mountain is very beneficial during the later stages of pregnancy, especially if you have numbness or a fluid build-up in your hands from carpal tunnel syndrome.

Trish, a friend of mine, used the Mountain to great benefit during the later part of her labour to help slow down the contractions and to give relief from the intense pressure she was feeling in the perineum. See chapter 21, Birth stories.

1. Rest on your hands and knees. Have your knees the same distance apart as your shoulders and your hands directly under your shoulders.
2. When you are ready, straighten your legs by lifting your hips upwards and gently ease your heels towards the

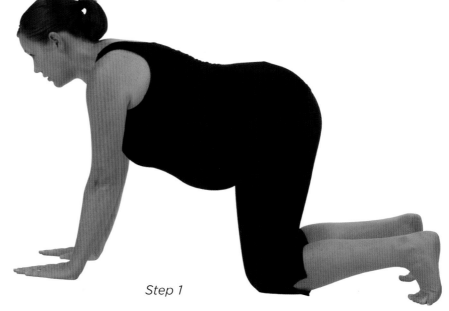

Step 1

floor. Hang your head in a relaxed way from your shoulders so that the muscles of your neck remain loose and relaxed. When you are in this posture, feel as if your hips are being drawn back towards your heels to feel the stretch in your back and spinal column and that the weight is more on your legs than your hands and arms. Hold the posture for the length of time that suits you best, remembering to breathe quietly and naturally.

To gain relief from the deep stretch in the backs of your legs, lift your heels away from the floor from time to time or return to your knees until you are ready to continue with the posture. Remember not to remain in the stretch if you are feeling discomfort in your legs or fullness in your face.

3. On completion, return to your knees and then relax in the Child Pose, either with your head resting on your hands or with your arms stretched out in front of you.

Alternative

Stand a little away from the wall with your feet hip-distance apart. Place your hands on the wall or on a window ledge and lower yourself down so that your torso comes to a horizontal position. This can be modified or extended to suit your

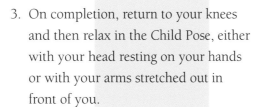

individual needs. Stretch back towards the legs so that you will feel a deep stretch in the hamstrings and throughout the back. Nearly everyone enjoys this and even those who like the Mountain find this is an excellent addition to their yoga practices. The benefits for your back and legs are similar and this position seems to effectively relieve tension in the shoulders.

This is a good alternative to the Mountain if you have high or low blood pressure, don't like having your head down, or find it too strenuous. A more upright variation of this is often used during labour to relieve backache and to benefit from the effects of gravity.

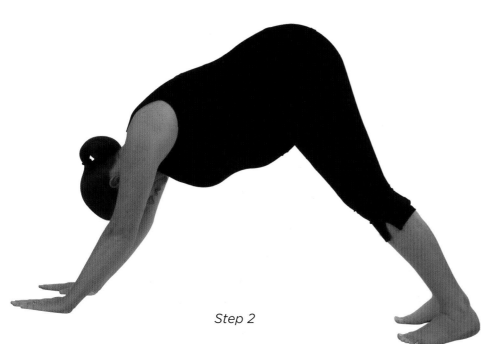

Step 2

CHAPTER 7

BALANCING POSTURES

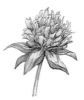

The balancing postures are an important part of any yoga program. Generally, they are not strenuous or demanding on the body, making them ideal for pregnancy and especially for someone who is a beginner to yoga. I recommend including at least one balancing posture in every yoga program, after first warming your body with some gentle stretches. There are other balancing postures, but these three are quite easy to do as well as being strengthening for the body.

During pregnancy your shape, size and weight are continually changing so it is important to be aware of your posture and carriage. Maintaining correct posture plays an important role in the prevention of backache, especially during the later months. If you look in a mirror side-on, you will be able to see whether you are standing correctly or are developing a sway or arch in the middle to lower back. The more regularly the balancing postures are practised the better your posture will be and the more poise and grace you will maintain.

As your balancing ability improves so will your general concentration and alertness, enabling you to remain focused without your mind wandering or losing your balance. This enhanced alertness and concentration supports a sense of inner calmness. Nervous tension is removed and a feeling of stillness and quietness is experienced. When these postures are done in sequence, you will notice your energies being drawn into a central point of awareness that is steady and focused. This is a similar feeling experienced during meditation.

The most difficult aspect of these postures is learning to stand on one leg with full breath and body awareness, without losing your balance. Gazing at a nearby stationary object will help steady your concentration and keep you from losing your balance. I suggest you also count your breaths, as this is an effective way of keeping your mind focused and helps you hold the posture for the same length of time on each side.

Keep the supporting foot and leg relaxed to alleviate tension and rigidity in your stance. You will also find balancing on one leg easier if your toes are spread evenly across the floor. Gripping the floor with your toes causes tension in the muscles of your feet and results in less floor contact.

The Tree: *Vriksasana*

The Tree is a classic balancing posture, very simple yet full of grace and merit. Physically, your supporting leg becomes stronger, your hip and thigh become more flexible and your knee is 'opened' out to the side.

This posture was practised by the yogis of India thousands of years ago. They were known to stand in this position for many days, deep in meditation. If you were to visit the holy city of Varanasi, on the sacred River Ganges, you might see this very thing happening today.

The Tree

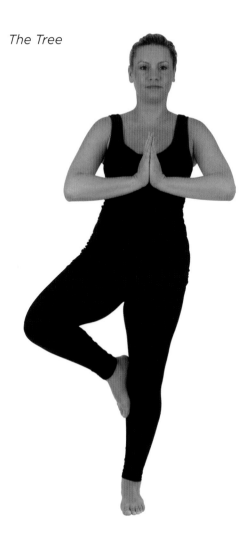

The Dynamic Tree

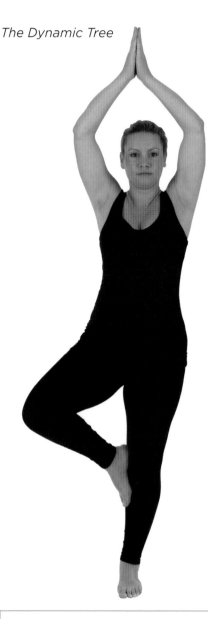

3. Place your right foot high on the inside of your left thigh. If your ankle is supple enough you can place your foot in front of your thigh, in the Half Lotus position (see page 92). Either way, your knee is taken out to the side, which encourages your hip to open. You will feel a deep stretch throughout your inner thigh and pelvic area.

4. Join your hands together at the centre of your chest in the prayer position. Keep your shoulders relaxed. Hold the final position for five breaths or longer if you wish.

5. Lower your foot to the floor and lightly shake your legs and feet.

6. Repeat the posture standing on your right leg, remembering always to hold the posture for the same amount of time on both sides.

The Dynamic Tree

The Tree practised with your arms raised above your head becomes the Dynamic Tree. From this position a full stretch is felt in the sides of your body and throughout your spinal column. Some people find balancing easier with their arms above their head, as it gives them a sense of being tall and steady. You might like to imagine an invisible cord running from the heel of your supporting foot right through the crown of your head and beyond to your fingertips, stretching your spine and holding you tall and straight. Hold the position for the same number of breaths on both sides.

1. Begin by standing with your feet a little apart and your body relaxed.

2. Choose a stationary object at eye level to focus on. When you are ready, rest your right foot on top of your left foot. You may wish to remain in this position until you gain confidence and your balance improves before lifting your leg to the traditional position. The point of this exercise is to balance on one leg, not where your raised leg is positioned.

Note: When practising the Tree do not 'sit down' into your hip by resting your weight on it as you might have seen photos of nomadic people doing, but lift up through your leg so that the sides of your body are straight, and your body is tall and erect.

The Eagle: *Garudasana*

This posture was named after the mythical Garuda, who was half man, half eagle and said to be the vehicle for the Hindu god, Vishnu. The eagle is king among birds and the possessor of great power and strength.

The benefits from practising the Eagle apply to both upper body and lower body. In the upper body, a deep stretch is felt in shoulders, upper arms, hands and fingers, and across the upper back. This movement is very useful for removing stiffness and tension in those areas and is especially beneficial for people with arthritis or rheumatism.

In the lower body the hips, thighs, knees and ankles are deeply toned, improving circulation and nerve tone. It is an excellent posture when leg cramps and sciatica are a problem. It also plays an important role in relieving varicose veins.

With your upper legs tightly crossed and your body bent slightly forward, your pelvic floor and lower body are nourished with a replenished blood supply. The further forward you bend and feel a deep 'squeezing' into your pelvic area, the more intense will be the benefits. However, I do not recommend you hold your body forward and squeeze tightly after the second or third month of pregnancy but instead use a more upright position. The benefits will still be felt without applying too much pressure to your pelvic area.

1. Begin by standing with your body straight and your focus on a stationary object.

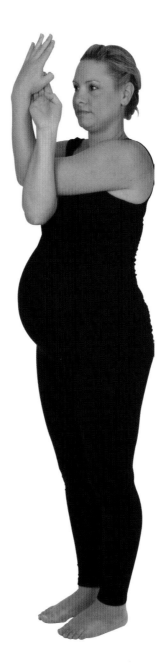

2. Extend your arms out in front of you at shoulder height. Cross your left arm over your right arm above your elbows or as high up your arms as possible. In this position you will feel a deep stretch across your back and your shoulders.

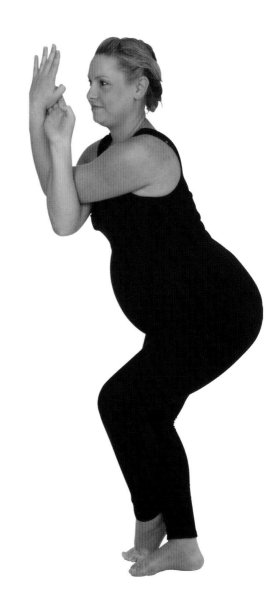

3. Bend your elbows and fold your arms inwards with your palms facing each other. Draw your arms in towards your body joining your fingers and palms. Hold your hands in front of your face and your arms close to your body.

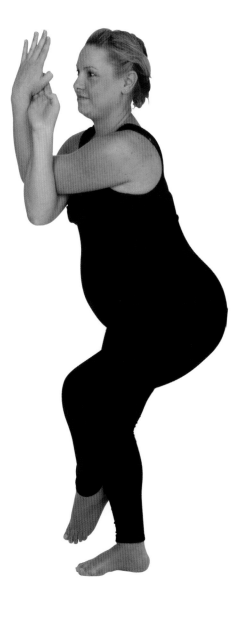

4. Bend your knees slightly as you cross your left leg over your right leg, so they are tightly squeezed at the upper thigh. Place the toes of your left foot on the floor beside your right foot. If you find balancing difficult this is a good alternative as you are still in the correct position and receiving all the benefits other than those from balancing. When you are steady the left foot is lifted off the floor and placed beside the right calf muscle.

5. Lean your body a little forward over your legs, 'sitting down' into the position and squeezing gently into your pelvic area. Hold the final posture and relax your breathing for five breaths.

6. When you are ready, come out of the posture. Breathe in while unfolding your arms and legs. Shake your legs and arms before repeating the exercise with your right arm and right leg crossing over your left, reversing all the movements and completing the posture on both sides.

Always take into account how you feel while practising the Eagle and adjust your position to suit your size and stage of pregnancy. The full Eagle, where the foot is taken toward the back of the calf muscle, is not recommended if you have swollen feet or are carrying excess fluid in your legs.

CHAPTER 8

PELVIC FLOOR EXERCISES

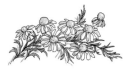

The pelvic floor exercises are one of the most important groups of exercises that all women should practise regularly, not only during pregnancy and after birth but throughout their lives. The demands on the muscles and ligaments of the pelvic floor are far greater during pregnancy and childbirth than at any other time in a woman's life. Just as other parts of the body are toned through regular exercise, so are the pelvic floor muscles. These simple exercises are an effective way of keeping these muscles strong and preventing problems developing later in life. Regular practice during pregnancy is essential, and they play an equally significant role after the birth in helping to restore firmness and strength.

In simple terms, the pelvic floor is a layer of overlapping and interconnecting muscles which extend from your pubic bone at the front, to your tail bone at the back and across the seat of your pelvic bone from one side to the other. Within this floor of muscles are three openings that lead to your pelvic organs; at the front is the urethra, leading to the bladder, the vagina in the centre leads to uterus, and the anus at the back leads to the rectum and large intestine. These muscles help to support your pelvic organs and your abdominal organs. Within the pelvic floor muscles are the sphincters, or ring-shaped muscles, of the bladder and your bowel, whose purpose is to help control bowel movements and the flow of urine. If your pelvic floor muscles are weak, or if these sphincters have lost their elasticity, incontinence can occur. There is a natural pressure on this group of muscles due to gravity and from bearing down when emptying the bladder and bowel. During pregnancy the pressure is obviously far greater due to increased body weight and increased blood volume.

Even women who do not have a vaginal delivery, or have never been pregnant, should exercise the pelvic floor on a daily basis well before the child-bearing years and for the rest of their lives. These exercises strengthen and tone the muscles of the pelvic area and the lower back, and are especially valuable where weakness is a problem in these areas. They are also an important group of exercises for men, due to their influence on the prostate and bladder.

Pelvic floor exercises are very important in preparation for birth. During the delivery it is important to know how to control the pelvic floor muscles so they can be relaxed and contracted when required. The more relaxed these muscles are, the easier the delivery will be and encourages women to be open and relaxed to birth their baby. The more children a woman has the greater care she will need to take of her pelvic floor muscles so that they stay firm and toned.

The pelvic floor exercises will help support and tone deeply into your vaginal and cervical areas. Some women are unaware of the very real possibility of post-birth incontinence, and it can be distressing and very embarrassing to find that even a sneeze, a cough or light jogging causes leakage from the bladder. If you realise you are already weak in these areas, continued practice will rectify the problem and help prevent incontinence later on.

These exercises tighten your anal muscles as well, which assists in preventing such problems as constipation and haemorrhoids. They also help overcome the possibility of anal and uterine prolapse, situations more common later in life. The subject of prolapse is not often talked about, but once it occurs it can be very difficult to reverse, often requiring medical intervention, so it is important to think about prevention early in life. In the past, lack of knowledge and education contributed to the development of these problems during the child-bearing years. Today, the situation is addressed in most antenatal classes and there is more open discussion among women and between women and their doctors.

How Are Pelvic Floor Exercises Done?

These exercises are simple enough to do, and can be practised anywhere and anytime without anyone knowing you are doing them. If you have a tendency to forget, choose a time and make a routine of it. I suggest during breakfast or morning or afternoon tea, every day, then it just becomes a good habit. This is probably a better option than when you're sitting at traffic lights—there's every chance that you will get green all the way or that you might not go out for a day or two. If you make a conscious effort to do them at a specific time of the day you will soon enjoy an increased strength, firmness and support. It has been suggested that they are a great asset to your sex life too.

Some people find it difficult to know when they are actually contracting the pelvic floor muscles and whether the 'lift' is enough. I suggest that you stop the flow of urine mid-flow when emptying your bladder, as it is your pelvic floor muscles that are being contracted when you do this. This only needs to be done once to correctly identify the muscles involved.

The position you use to do the exercises is a personal choice, but some positions make it easier to identify the muscles involved and whether you are doing the exercises correctly. Some women find they have more awareness from a standing position leaning slightly forward; others notice the sensation more when sitting, others in the Butterfly posture. As you progress through your pregnancy you might need to change position due to the weight of your uterus. If you are carrying low, leaning forward from a standing or kneeling position takes the weight away from the pelvic floor slightly so the feeling is more obvious.

1. Gently tighten and hold your perineum and pelvic floor without ever feeling contraction in the abdominal area. Lift deeply enough to feel the tightening in your urethra, lower bowel and vagina.
2. Hold the contraction to the count of five, and then slowly release and relax the muscles. Some women like to think of going up and down in an elevator, but do whatever is easiest for you and the most effective.
3. This exercise can be repeated as many times as you like but as a general guide practise contracting your muscles ten times, three times a day.

Some authorities suggest 100 repetitions a day, or more, which can be a daunting thought, but this recommendation does come from experts in this field. Setting a reasonable number in your mind to begin with is better than being overwhelmed and doing none at all. Once you have established a regular routine gradually increase the number. After the birth continue to practise them on a daily basis.

Breathing and Humming with the Pelvic Floor Exercises

Women are often quite reluctant to do these exercises which in the past has been a concern to me, even when 'horror stories' were told with the purpose of spurring them into regular practice. When I included breathing and/or humming in conjunction with the exercises, I found that women often enjoyed them more and

better understood why they were doing them and their value.

To add breathing, contract your pelvic floor muscles while breathing in, then release the hold as you breathe out through the mouth. The outgoing breath is always associated with release and relaxation, especially when it is done through the mouth. This is important for the birth, for when you have your mind firmly in that part of the body, and are breathing relaxation into it, your whole attention is where it needs to be. This means that physically and mentally you are helping the perineum to relax and the cervix to open—you are consciously helping yourself and your baby through each moment of labour to birth. The mouth being open as you breathe out encourages the facial muscles to be relaxed, and relates to the cervix being relaxed and open too.

As you do these exercises with your breathing your awareness is on being soft, open and relaxed. This concept is important when labour begins as it encourages you to go with the contractions rather than tightening up against them. It is a natural response to withdraw from pain and discomfort, to tighten the body and even attempt to remove or distract yourself mentally from the intensity of labour. However, the more you have your mind on breathing into the sensations, to open and relax consciously as well as physically, the more positive you will stay which encourages you to

trust in yourself and have confidence that it is possible for birth to be a wonderful experience.

Humming, discussed fully on page 103, can also be done in conjunction with the pelvic floor exercises. Many women have found this to be very centring, grounding and internalising as a birth preparation and a valuable asset during the birth that encourages you to realise the potential of your thoughts and the purpose of your breath. Breathe in and tighten the pelvic floor muscles and focus on drawing energy and prana into this part of your body. As you breathe out and hum, relax the muscles and direct the 'sound' and the vibration into the pelvic floor. This is a powerful birth preparation practice and can be done throughout pregnancy—and in the last weeks before the birth also imagine the cervix softening in preparation for birth as you hum and exhale.

As you inhale you might like to repeat an empowering affirmation or even a single word which is then carried with the breath and with the healing sound, for example, 'open', or 'relax'. It is possible to hum with your mouth a little open by resting your tongue against the soft palate so that your mouth and jaw are relaxed.

Moola Bandha and *Ashwini Mudra*

The pelvic floor exercises can be compared to the yoga practices *moola bandha* and *ashwini mudra*, which basically involve lifting, locking and tightening different parts of the pelvic floor.

Traditionally, *moola bandha* is included in the advanced yoga practice Tantra Yoga, which is based on awareness of the chakras. The Sanskrit word *moola* means 'root' or 'source'; *bandha* means to lock or tighten a specific part of your body. The nature of the practice is to lift, tighten and hold the muscles of your pelvic floor. When *moola bandha* is practised it is stimulating the base or root chakra, known as *mooladhara*, which is said to be located in your perineum or, more accurately, the perineum of a man and the cervical area of a woman. In some texts it is *ashwini mudra* which is likened to the pelvic floor exercises because it involves tightening the anus. I feel that the pelvic floor exercises are really a combination of the two practices, for both areas that are involved when you do them correctly. When you become skilled with the pelvic floor exercises you can isolate the two areas and practise tightening them separately.

The root chakra is an important point of meditation for pregnancy and birth, and a logical one, as I discuss in a chakra meditation on page 134. When *moola bandha* is practised regularly it is said to have a stimulating effect on the eyebrow centre chakra, ajna chakra, which is the area of the conscious mind and the pathway of greater awareness. I have noticed that as women continue with their yoga practices, in a very short time they become more aware and enjoy greater insight and wisdom. Although pregnant women naturally tend to become more intuitive and more internalised in the months leading up to the birth, and regular practice of yoga increases awareness, I wonder if there is another, more spiritually inclined benefit derived from practising the pelvic floor exercises. I include them in every class and encourage their practice every day.

CHAPTER 9

MUDRAS

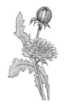

The Sanskrit word *mudra* means an attitude or gesture by a part of your body. It also refers to a part of your body that is sealed or closed off. In eastern dance, mudras are seen in the gestures of the hands, fingers and eyes which the dancer uses to represent specific moods and feelings.

Many of the mudras in yoga are quite involved, and only practised by experienced devotees; others are of the simplest nature, the modest positions of the fingers and the eyes recommended here.

The prominent yoga teacher, Swami Satyananda, says in *Yoga Nidra, Deep Relaxation*, that a mudra is: 'a psychic attitude often expressed by a physical gesture, movement or posture which affects the flow of psychic energy in the body'.

When these simple gestures are included with a yoga posture they have a subtle yet profound effect on mental and spiritual aspects. I recommend they be used during meditation, relaxation and while practising the breathing exercises. The hands are channels for the meridians in the body and because the hands are touching in the mudras, energy flow is continuous around the body.

Five mudras are especially relevant for pregnancy. The first four are generally used during meditation, deep relaxation or while practising the breathing exercises. The fifth, *shambhavi mudra*, is often considered part of advanced yoga practices but has important benefits during pregnancy, especially when done occasionally before the Candle Meditation (page 124).

The Psychic Gestures of Consciousness and Knowledge: *Chin Mudra* and *Gyana Mudra*

Chin mudra and *gyana mudra* are very similar and their benefits are also comparable. Although they are very simple to do their influence is profound, and at the same time subtle. It may not be immediately apparent that they are quietening your mind, but with time and patience your awareness will become finely tuned to their delicate energies.

According to traditional yogic texts, the index finger represents the soul and the thumb represents higher or supreme consciousness. In joining them an important connection is made between your soul and your higher consciousness or spiritual energy. The union of your psychic mind and physical nervous system causes impulses from your hands to be

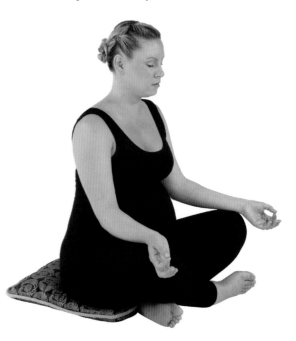

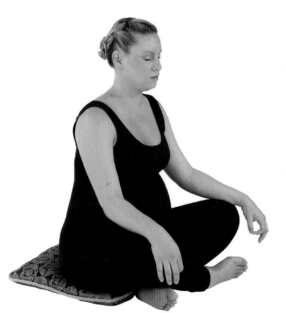

or annulment of the universe, but in practice it is a very soft and unassuming way of holding your hands. Like the first two mudras, it encourages a peaceful feeling.

Sit in a comfortable position with your spine straight and your body relaxed. With both palms facing upwards, place your right hand on top of your left. The left hand on top of the right hand is known as *bhairavi mudra*, which is the female equivalent of *bhairava mudra*. With your hands resting at the base of your belly, this mudra gives a lovely sense that you are holding your baby gently in your womb.

Dhyani mudra, the gesture of meditation, is very similar—the left hand rests in the right hand with the thumb tips touching.

The Womb or Source: *Yoni Mudra*

Yoni mudra has particular relevance for women, especially during pregnancy, as the word *yoni* means 'womb' or 'source'. In Barbara Walker's massive tome, *The Woman's Encyclopaedia of Myths and Secrets*, yoni is described as 'the Primordial Image representing the Great Mother as the source of all life'. Walker goes on: 'as the genital focus of her divine energy, the Yoni Yantra was adorned as a geometrical symbol, as the cross was adorned by Christians'. *Yantra* refers to a symbolic shape used for concentration and meditation, or the visual aspect of a mantra or spiritual sound. The *yoni yantra* is a downward-facing triangle; the hands in *yoni mudra* represent a downward-facing triangle, which is seen at the centre of the traditional symbol for the base chakra.

directed back into your body as prana, or psychic energy. You might find yourself intuitively joining your thumb and first finger during your quieter yoga practices.

Sit in a comfortable position and place your hands on your knees. Join the tips of your thumb and index finger, on each hand. Your other fingers will naturally curl slightly inwards. For *chin mudra*, your palms face up; for *gyana mudra* your palms face down.

For deep relaxation (yoga nidra), use *chin mudra*.

The Terrifying Attitude: *Bhairava Mudra*

Bhairava mudra is a comfortable and easy way to hold your hands for the breathing exercises, meditation or while resting. The name refers to the fierce or terrifying attitude of Lord Shiva and the separation

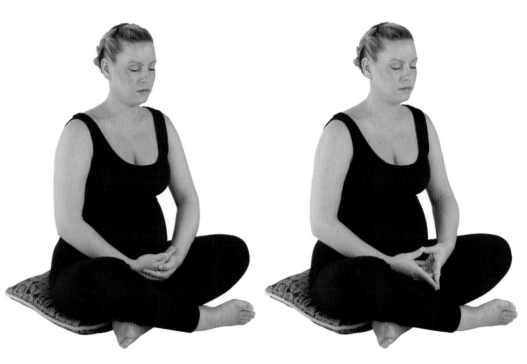

Yoni mudra will bring quietness and stillness to your mind and body in a most powerful way and also bring balance the left and right sides of your brain. It is excellent to use when practising your yoga breathing and while meditating, because it helps to intensify concentration as well as deep relaxation.

Yoni mudra is the mudra most preferred by pregnant women—maybe because they are intuitively drawn to its deep symbolism but also because the arms and shoulders are relaxed when the hands are held in this way and is therefore relaxing for the whole upper body.

1. Sit in a comfortable position with your spine straight, your eyes lightly closed and your body and mind relaxed.
2. With your arms relaxed and your hands resting in your lap, interlock your fingers. Spread your hands slightly, straighten your index fingers and join the tips together, and do the same with the tips of the thumbs. Your fingers pointing downwards form a downward-facing triangle symbolising the *yoni yantra* and the entrance to the womb.

Eyebrow Centre Gazing:
Shambhavi Mudra

Shambhavi mudra is one of the most powerful yoga practices for accessing the more peaceful aspects of the inner mind and ultimately the higher consciousness, and therefore an important preparation for all meditations. It has a quietening effect on your mind and induces a more inward perception, encouraging us to recognise a quieter place within ourselves. *Shambhavi mudra* induces a deep calmness and restfulness in the mind so that emotional stability is gradually improved and concentration is also benefited. With regular practice your eyes and the muscles around your eyes will become stronger.

1. Sit in a comfortable cross-legged position, or in your bean bag. Use any one of the hand mudras and close your eyes lightly.
2. Open your eyes and focus on a point in front of you. Your head can be tilted back slightly for comfort. Look up towards your eyebrows and then draw your focus in to the point at the centre of your eyebrows. Keep

your face and eyes relaxed and blink if you need to and when you are ready close your eyes. If you feel any strain or discomfort, close your eyes immediately.

3. Keep your eyes closed for a short time and then repeat the practice. At first it might be a little uncomfortable to hold this position for any length of time, but with practice it becomes easier and your eyes can be held open for longer. When you close your eyes you will notice a feeling of calmness and stillness in your mind. Some people refer to it as a vast open space, as if you are being drawn into the most peaceful part of your inner consciousness.

Shambhavi mudra is part of an advanced yoga study called Kriya Yoga and is one of the main practices for stimulating and awakening *ajna chakra*, the eyebrow centre chakra. If you wish to explore this more deeply it is preferable to seek the assistance of a proficient teacher.

CHAPTER 10

SEATED POSTURES FOR PRANAYAMA AND MEDITATION

If you create an auspicious condition in your body and your environment, the meditation and realisation will automatically arise.

Sogyal Rinpoche, *Meditation*, page 32

Sitting on the floor for any length of time can be a new experience and sometimes quite uncomfortable, but with a little patience you will find some of the postures recommended here can be managed and maintained in complete comfort. To obtain the full benefit from your meditation practice it is paramount that you are completely comfortable in your position, especially as your pregnancy progresses. If you don't find any of the four postures to your liking you might prefer to sit in a three-quarters filled bean bag.

It is also acceptable to sit on cushions to help overcome initial discomfort. Placing one or two small cushions under your tail bone will elevate your lower body and tilt your pelvis slightly forward, allowing your knees to rest closer to the floor enabling you to sit with your spine straight and back relaxed for the duration of the practice. The cushions will help relieve discomfort, especially in your lower back. This elevated position also gives some extra room at the top of the abdomen if you are carrying high. A bean bag provides the same elevation to your pelvis as well as added support for your back.

The first four postures are traditionally used for the breathing exercises and meditation. If you are going to try them, begin with the easiest and most comfortable position. The fifth posture, the Breath Balancing posture, can be done from any position where you are relaxed and your spine is straight.

Spending a little time each day in the easier postures will quickly increase your flexibility and in time you can include the more challenging postures if you choose. The main aim is to be able to hold a posture comfortably and not be distracted by your body, without changing your position unless you really have to. In the early days of learning to meditate it is normal to feel discomfort in various parts of your body, including your legs, ankles, back and shoulders, and for your feet to go to sleep occasionally. This is why the positions recommended here are simply a guideline—your comfort is what will make a difference to your enjoyment and the benefits you receive from the meditations, not your posture.

In all these postures it is important to hold your spine as straight as possible and to keep your body completely relaxed. Generally, your eyes are lightly closed, your teeth a little apart and your face soft and relaxed. Keep your arms slightly bent at the elbows to prevent tension in your arms and shoulders. I recommend that your hands be resting in one of the mudras from the previous chapter, but if you prefer you can rest your hands on your abdomen. Before sitting remember to loosen your feet and hips with a few ankle exercises, and/or the hip rotation or the Butterfly.

The Easy Posture: *Sukhasana*

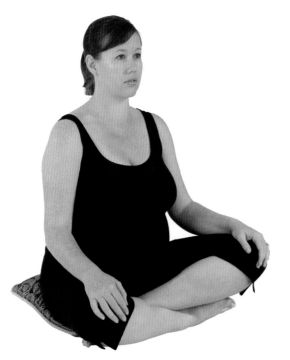

Sitting on the floor with your legs crossed may appear easy, but unless it's a regular habit you might find it very uncomfortable to begin with. With regular practice the Easy Posture often becomes a favourite, especially with beginners.

In this easy position your body will feel steady and balanced and your mind calm and settled, so important for enjoying the benefits from pranayama and meditation. Your back and spinal column feel firm and strong—sometimes it is helpful to imagine you have space between each vertebra to give a feeling of lightness in the spine. With practice your knees, ankles and hips become flexible and loose and the pelvic area becomes more open and supple.

1. Begin by sitting with your legs stretched out in front of you.
2. Bend your right leg and place your right foot under your left thigh. Place your left foot under your right thigh. Adjust your position until you are completely comfortable, then close your eyes. This posture can be held for as long as desired. When you have completed the practice, unfold your legs and shake them lightly.

The Adept's Posture: *Siddhasana*

In this posture your knees will come closer to the floor than in the Easy Posture and with practice most people can manage it easily. The benefits are similar to the previous posture, with more flexibility encouraged in your hips and pelvis.

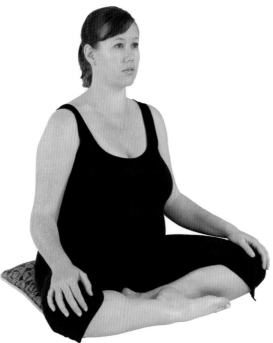

1. Begin in the Easy Posture, then pull your left heel in against your perineum or as close to your pelvic floor as possible.
2. Place your right heel in front of your left ankle and feel relaxed in your whole body.

The Half Lotus and Full Lotus

These more challenging positions are not suitable for everyone, nor always of interest, but as they are so important in traditional yoga they are worth attempting, especially if you are a dedicated student. They are considered the most appropriate and advantageous postures for deep meditation and, ultimately, sense withdrawal. In the Lotus the practitioner comes to realise increased mental clarity and emotional calmness. This results in detachment from passing thoughts, allowing you to simply witness the movement of your thoughts with a quiet awareness, in the same way the breath is observed as it moves freely in and out of the body.

With practice stiffness is removed from your knees, hips and ankles and circulation is improved to your lower back and pelvis. As there is a greater blood supply to your abdominal area, this posture is also beneficial for your digestive system and reproductive system. Your spine is encouraged to remain upright and steady which creates the correct atmosphere for the flow of prana up and down your spinal column.

It is important to practise these postures in a gentle manner and never experience pain or extreme discomfort in the final position. These postures are important, but not as important as the meditation practices or skill with your breathing exercises. To obtain the most benefits from them, ensure you are comfortable so you can relax and when ever possible that your spine is held straight.

Before commencing these postures, loosen and relax your feet and your ankles by practising the ankle exercises, hip rotations, the Butterfly or the squatting exercises.

The Half Lotus: *Ardha Padmasana*

Ardha padmasana means 'half lotus', and is a good preparation for the Lotus posture. It is best practised when the easier seated postures have been mastered and can be maintained for the duration of your meditation.

Sit with your legs in front of you. Place your left foot on top of your right thigh. Rest your right foot beside your left inner thigh, as close to your groin as possible. This can be reversed to gain flexibility in both ankles and legs. Lightly close your eyes and hold the posture for as long as you are comfortable. When you release your legs from the posture, shake them lightly.

The Lotus: *Padmasana*

This highly recognisable posture is one of the most important in traditional yogic teachings. For many it is the posture of choice for meditation and advanced pranayama; once mastered it brings balance and stability to both mind and body. It is not the easiest of postures to become accustomed to but with regular practice and dedication the final position will be achieved. I recommend you practise the Half Lotus and feel comfortable in that posture before attempting the Lotus.

1. Sit on the floor with your legs in front of you and your spine straight.
2. Bend your right leg and place your right foot on top of your left thigh, as close to your groin as possible.
3. Bend your left leg and place your left foot on your right thigh. Move your knees as close to the floor as possible. Your heels need to be as close as possible to your pelvis with the soles of your feet facing upward. Close your eyes and relax into your meditation. When you release your legs from the posture, shake them lightly.

At no time force your legs into the Lotus posture. Many yoga postures are new to your body, and it takes time and patience for the muscles to become free and loose enough to achieve them comfortably. Some people are naturally very flexible and can easily manage all the yoga postures, whereas others are limited by lesser flexibility or the result of injury.

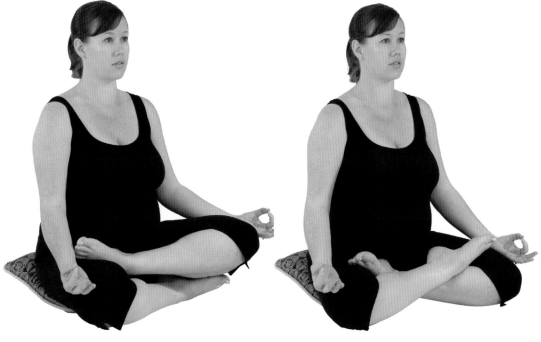

The Breath Balancing Posture: *Padadhirasana*

It is quite natural for one nostril to be easier to breathe through than the other and this becomes more obvious during the breathing exercises discussed in the next chapter, especially Alternate Nostril breathing. The Breath Balancing pose is a simple and very effective way to equalise the flow of the breath through the nostrils and bring a peaceful atmosphere to the mind. This is because there are pressure points under the armpits that correspond to the sinuses and by placing gentle finger pressure under the armpits the flow of the breath through the nostrils can be equalised, or at the least improved. When the fingers of the left hand are placed high in the right armpit the left nostril is eventually cleared, and the same applies in

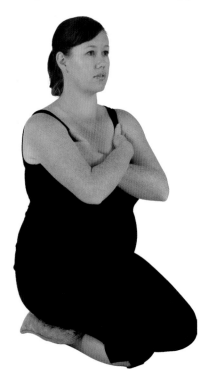

reverse. When the breath is equal through both nostrils you are more relaxed and calm and both sides of your brain are balanced. I might mention that the left nostril corresponds to the right side of the brain, the feminine part, and the right nostril to the left side of the brain, the masculine part.

It is interesting to be aware of which nostril is clear when you are relaxed and your mind is calm. Most probably it will be your left nostril, as it corresponds to the quieter and less analytical right side of your brain, or the feminine side. This is worthwhile remembering when you are having trouble sleeping—if you lie on your right side, the flow of air will be increased in your left nostril and stimulate the right side of your brain, helping you to relax. On the other hand, if you need to 'wake up' or think more clearly, then it is your right nostril which needs to be flowing freely so that the left brain is more 'awake'.

Any time you need to be still and centred, the Breath Balancing posture will very quickly and gently help to establish a quieter atmosphere in your mind. It can be combined with most of your breathing exercises and meditations. You might have noticed people in conversation with their arms crossed over their chest in this manner. Some would say it is body language suggesting protection or covering of the heart centre. This may be true, but I feel it is because we know instinctively that when we have our arms crossed in

this way we are relaxed and balanced and therefore more likely to have a calm and pleasant conversation.

1. Sit in a comfortable position with your spine straight and your eyes lightly closed.
2. Cross your arms in front of your chest with your right arm in front of your left, and place your fingertips high up into your armpits. Keep your thumbs outside your armpits, facing up. Make sure your shoulders are soft and relaxed.
3. Concentrate on breathing quietly and stay in this posture for as long as desired. You will notice the longer you remain in this posture the slower your breathing becomes and the more relaxed you feel.

I suggest practising *ujjayi pranayama* (page 106) or humming while sitting in this posture because one practice really complements the other. When you are humming feel the lovely vibration and sound in your chest as your breathe out. With your hands in the Breath Balancing position it is easier to bring your awareness to the breath in your chest and to find comfort and relaxation in that, so that as well as bringing balance to the brain and calming the mind, this simple posture is an excellent meditation in itself. Used in the early moments of labour, the many benefits of the combination of these practices provide a way to stay present and focused.

CHAPTER 11
BREATHING EXERCISES: PRANAYAMA

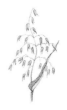

The yoga breathing exercises form a group of traditional techniques that are in many ways the most important aspect of your birth preparation. Your awareness of the breath, your ability to use the enormous potential within it and know how to breathe consciously will help you more than any other aspect of yoga as you move through labour. As you come to understand these simple yet excellent practices you will come to trust them and have faith in their worth, not only in childbirth but in your everyday life.

Pranayama relaxes and replenishes your physical body. It calms and balances your emotional self. It is nourishment for your mind through clarity and wisdom—and provides the opportunity to bring your attention to yourself, to your thoughts, the nature of your thoughts and the atmosphere they create in your mind. Mindfulness, concentration and purity of awareness. It also helps you to become more aware of your spiritual self, your soul—the ageless essence that brings life to all the other parts of you, that makes you who you are. Your breath is a constant companion, with you from the moment of birth until the moment you die. The breathing exercises provide the opportunity to simply be, to be alone and at peace with yourself. To watch the flow of the natural breath moving gently through your body holds you profoundly in the present moment, calm, steady and in complete consciousness.

The yoga breathing is the foundation of all yoga practices and yoga without it is not true yoga. Breath awareness is at the core of any meditation and relaxation practices you might explore. The beauty of breathing awareness is that is it always there for you, to bring your attention back to yourself, to bring your 'mind back home'. You don't need any external aid—it is with you every moment of your life.

The nature of your breath is a guide to your state of mind—if you are relaxed it will be unwavering and rhythmic, if you are feeling restless or anxious it is likely to be shallow and unsteady. Your knowledge of the yoga breathing practices will benefit you the most during the intensity of labour. Realistically, you won't be relaxing into a lovely spinal twist but understanding the breathing will help you to focus, to feel strong and courageous and to calm yourself. It will help you be there consciously with your body and your baby in your womb.

Life is the interval between one breath and another—he who only breathes half, only lives half. But he who masters the art of breathing has control over every function of his being.

Shri Yogendra, *Hatha Yoga Simplified*, page 17

The word *prana* means 'energy', 'vitality', 'wind', 'life force', 'respiration'. 'No greater element than bioenergy (*prana*) exists in the body,' says Shri Yogendra. The word *yama* means 'to control'. The practice of pranayama is to control or to influence the vital energy and life force that is within each and every breath. It also means being able to utilise this energy to its fullest capacity as it flows through the body and mind as you breathe. As you feel your breath in your body, know there is prana within it and draw on that to move with the energy of birth, to be there—present, positive, relaxed and strong.

Be conscious of that energy as you breathe and become one with the breath so you are in meditation with it. Be completely aware of every moment of the inhalation and how your body moves with that, and with every moment of the exhalation feel and observe the breath gently and quietly leaving your body. Breath awareness means you are conscious in that moment and totally present. One-pointed awareness on the breath is the first step to mindfulness and meditation. It is a meditation in itself.

Breathing is a completely natural process that is mostly unconscious. Through the practice of pranayama we gradually become more aware of the movements of our breath, witnessing and observing its rhythmic, steady flow in and out of the body. Pranayama is so vital to our wellbeing that to practise yoga without it is to realise only a fraction its true potential.

When we breathe more efficiently it ensures a healthy blood flow to the brain, which encourages the mind to be clear and steady, and more likely to be free from mental confusion. During moments of stress, breathing usually becomes faster, shallower and higher in the chest. This means less oxygen is circulating around the body and reaching the brain, creating a stress cycle that results in diminished clarity and sometimes confused or irrational behaviour.

But if we can distance ourselves from the stressful moment, witness the way we are breathing and remember to breathe slowly, steadily and consciously, we can create a space for clearer and more logical thinking. We will then be more relaxed and present and better able to manage our response to the stress. Of course, this is often easier said than done, but it can be done when we are skilled with the breathing exercises and understand their many benefits.

One of the main purposes of pranayama is to bring about feelings of quietness and stillness in the mind. Over time, you will become more skilled with the practices, and others will notice a difference in your nature as you become a little more relaxed, and your life somehow seems less hectic—where you realise it is possible to be calm amid the chaos. Just as it is essential to exercise the body, it is equally important to discipline ourselves to breathe more efficiently and with awareness. It provides the space in a busy life to know yourself a little better, to find contentment in some quiet time alone, at peace with yourself.

Preparation for Pranayama

You will gain the most from practising pranayama when you are aware of the following points:

1. If at all possible, begin pranayama exercises under the guidance of an experienced teacher, so that if problems arise they can be quickly corrected.

2. Always proceed slowly and gradually. If you feel light-headed or faint, stop the exercise immediately until you feel better and have restored balance in your breathing. This is not a common problem, but can occur when the breathing is not steady and even, or when deep yoga breathing is repeated too often. Correct breathing is always equal, so that what you breathe in is the same as you breathe out.

3. The traditional seated postures are described in the previous chapter. If you find them hard to manage you can sit with your back against a wall, on cushions if required, with your legs straight out in front, or sit in a straight-backed chair with your legs uncrossed and your feet flat on the floor. Many pregnant women prefer to sit in a bean bag. If you can manage a crossed-leg position use one or two cushions for support. Your spine should always be as straight as possible and your body relaxed. If your baby is in the posterior position it is important to resist leaning back, whether you are practising your breathing and meditation or watching TV. Stay as upright as possible using cushions for the support you need.

4. Whenever you do your yoga asanas or other exercises, leave some time for the breathing practices too. They can be

practised after the asanas and before meditation and relaxation. They are an excellent way to calm the mind in preparation for meditation and greatly enhance the quality of your meditation practice. If you are feeling distressed or exhausted they can be practised on their own for very positive results. There is no time limit on how long you should practise pranayama—sometimes 10 minutes is enough—but if you are unsettled or restless 20 minutes or more will bring the results you most want.

5. To begin with, allow about 10 minutes for pranayama. Over time this can be increased to meet your specific needs. Keep each breath flowing evenly and smoothly in and out of your body—never 'jerking' your breathing or rushing. At no time become breathless or short of breath. Remember not to strain your breathing in an effort to complete an exercise, always keeping in mind that the practices are gentle

---

Caution: Deep breathing is not recommended for people with high blood pressure or heart problems. If your doctor approves, proceed by slow degrees and under experienced supervision so that your body becomes accustomed to these practices gently and safely.

---

and designed to have a calming and relaxing effect on all levels.

6. During pregnancy it is not advisable to hold your breath but rather to keep your breath flowing evenly through your body. A short breath retention, known as *kumbhaka*, is acceptable when you are proficient with the breathing practices, but this needs to be taught under the guidance of an experienced teacher and only when you are competent with all other aspects of pranayama.

7. Your body needs to be completely relaxed and free of tension. Have your eyes lightly closed, your teeth a little apart and your jaw relaxed. Your hands can be placed on your knees, on your abdomen or in one of the mudras (page 88). Have your arms slightly bent to prevent tension building up in arms and shoulders.

8. Before you begin your breathing exercises, practise the Heavenly Stretch posture (page 69) and some of the other exercises where your chest is expanded such as the shoulder rotations (page 67). This reduces tension in the upper body, encourages more efficient breathing and prepares your lungs.

9. Practise in a well-ventilated room, away from outside disturbances and distracting noises. If you can, take the phone off the hook and let others know you would appreciate some quiet time on your own.

10. Wear loose comfortable clothing. Your body temperature will drop as you become more relaxed, so it is useful to cover your shoulders with a light rug before you begin and wear socks in cooler weather.

11. If possible, practise before eating. This is not always practical during pregnancy, especially if you are having fluctuations in your blood sugar levels or suffer from nausea. A snack of almonds, pecan nuts, sunflower seeds and pumpkin seeds is better than a full meal.

12. Before you start, spend a few quiet moments following your natural breath and clearing your mind so that you feel calm and centred.

Always be mindful that the incoming breath is there to supply you with the qualities and energies you need to maintain balance and harmony on all levels. The outgoing breath is about releasing tension and stress from body and mind, to help you to relax. In this way you are using the breath and your thoughts to create the feelings most needed at the time. This is conscious breathing.

The Natural Breath

Although the natural breath is not a breathing exercise as such, it is in many ways the most important breath to understand and feel comfortable with. It is also the starting point for all the other practices. When you are one with the breath, you are present, mindful and calm.

It is natural for the mind to wander, but knowing how to centre your mind through simple breath awareness is an effective way to witness the gap between your thoughts and be there in the present moment. Although the interval between one thought and the next might be brief, focusing on gentle breathing enables you to hold your attention steady, to observe the preciousness of the moment now, and to be alone and at peace with yourself. Life is transient and much of the time it flashes by without our full conscious attention. When you bring your attention to your natural breath, you are there, totally present and living your life in that moment.

So following your natural breath is where to begin, watching the movement of your breath as it gently flows in and out of your body. The more you practise this, the more strength of mind you will develop, and the greater confidence you will feel in yourself. Some find it easier to feel the movement of the breath in their abdomen, others feel it more in the chest, just watching it as it softly rises and falls in the body. When you have a comforting association with breath awareness, as soon as you focus on breathing you will feel calm and relaxed—and also strong and together. You can do this anywhere and at any time. From this basic breath awareness you can move into the other breathing practices, and to meditation. Interestingly, one of the most profound meditations is

simply observing the rhythmic, constant movement of the breathing—so simple yet centring and grounding.

I suggest counting the breaths, in groups of five or more, in and out of the nose, or in through the nose and out through the mouth. Counting will help you to stay focused, stop your mind from wandering and improve concentration. This is conscious breathing, which gives you steadiness and clarity and a one pointed awareness on the breath.

If you are feeling exhausted you can energise yourself through drawing on the prana or energy within each breath and what you focus on as you inhale. You can breathe in and repeat an empowering word or phrase to bring about the feelings and energies you need. Even when this is done for a short time you will notice the benefits.

Witnessing your breathing is also the quickest way to relax during pregnancy and after the birth as well. As you count your breaths, focus on each one taking you deeper and deeper into a calm quiet space in your mind— where you are using your breathing and your thoughts to create a feeling of inner stillness.

When it is difficult to bring your mind to the breath, I suggest placing one hand on the abdomen and one on the chest so you can feel the parts of your body involved. If you find it easier to focus on the breath in the abdomen, place both hands there. The Breath Balancing Pose will give more emphasis to the breath in

your chest, or you might prefer to block your ears and listen to the gentle sound of your resting breath.

The Complete Yoga Breath or Deep Yoga Breathing

The value of the Complete Yoga Breath cannot be over-emphasised—the whole person benefits in a dynamic and positive way. Most people breathe in a very shallow manner where the breath is light and short within the chest cavity and the muscles of the chest and upper/middle back are never fully expanded. Before people learn to breathe from a yogic perspective they are generally not using the full capacity of their lungs and therefore have a much diminished uptake and utilisation of oxygen.

The middle of your body—or your solar plexus—is often referred to as the emotional centre of the physical body. When we are feeling unsettled emotionally, in times of fear, anxiety or anger this part of the body tightens, becomes tense and 'closes up'. We feel 'uncomfortable in the stomach', with nervous sensations often accompanied by nausea and cramping; if stress becomes chronic, digestive problems can result. This tightness through the solar plexus also affects the way we breathe and prevents correct abdominal breathing and therefore completion of a full yogic breath.

We can divide the cycle of a breath into inhalation, retention (which for pregnancy is kept to a minimum) and exhalation. The incoming and outgoing breaths should be equal in length. With regular practice your breathing will improve, as will your control of the breath. The breath becomes longer, deeper and slower, your lungs are encouraged to expand more completely, and the whole respiratory system strengthens and works more efficiently.

Abdominal Breathing

In abdominal breathing your abdomen is gently pushed out and the diaphragm lowers slightly to allow the base of your lungs to expand. To begin with, exaggerate this movement to really feel your abdominal area working. It can help to imagine a balloon in the abdomen that inflates and deflates as you breathe, with the emphasis on relaxing these muscles rather than drawing them inwards. If you place your fingertips together on your navel you will notice them move apart as you inhale and come together again as you exhale. When abdominal breathing is done correctly, your navel appears to move out as you breathe in and fall back into your body as you breathe out.

Abdominal breathing has many advantages especially in times of anxiety, panic attacks and confusion, and can be used if there is tightness or cramping in your abdomen or pelvic area. Being able to control the flow and depth of the breath is advantageous to restoring equilibrium in the breathing and encourage the right balance of oxygen and carbon dioxide, to re-establish clear thinking and a more rational response to stressful situations.

Relaxed deeper breathing can then follow.

Relaxed abdominal breathing is important during birthing, because the abdomen is where you will be feeling the contractions. By breathing with the focus on your abdomen, your attention will be held there. This will help you to relax into the contraction better and reduce pain caused by tight and tense muscles. It also

encourages you to be there with your baby as you move through the birthing process together. This is best done by breathing in through the nose and out through the mouth, with the emphasis on relaxing and releasing tensions and being ever mindful of softening, letting go and opening to the birth of your baby.

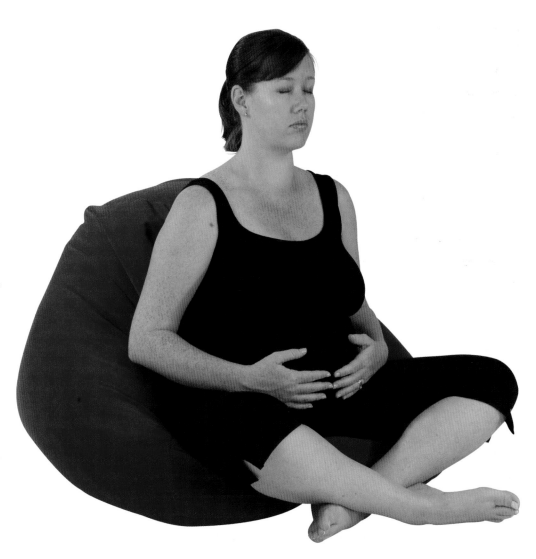

Thoracic Breathing

In thoracic breathing your breath is taken deeply into your upper chest for a full expansion of your chest. Your shoulders lift slightly and your whole upper body expands as your lungs push your rib cage wide. When you exhale, the muscles of your chest relax and contract, and your abdominal muscles relax and move back into your body. If your fingertips are placed together in the middle of your chest, you will notice them move slightly apart as you breathe in and come together again as you breathe out. The whole movement is slow and controlled without any strain or shortness of breath. You will notice the breath moving in your chest more easily with your hands in the Breath Balancing pose.

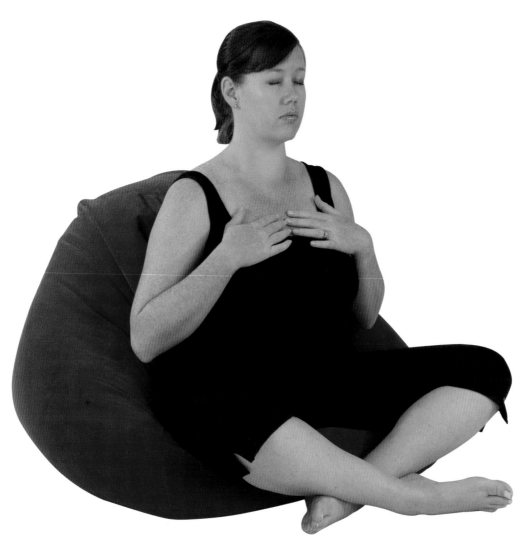

Deep Yoga Breathing

Here abdominal breathing and thoracic breathing are combined to make a slow full breath for a complete expansion and contraction of your lungs. Your body lifts and expands while breathing in, and contracts and relaxes as you breathe out.

As you begin to inhale your abdomen is expanded outwards, allowing your diaphragm to move down and the base of your lungs to expand. Your breath continues slowly to fill your middle and upper chest. When you breathe out, gently push the last remaining air from your lungs so that you feel your abdomen flatten slightly. I emphasise this point because sometimes people breathe in deeply but don't breathe out completely. Breathing in and out evenly maintains equilibrium throughout your body.

When you first practise deep yogic breathing I suggest no more than two or three breaths at a time, three times a day. As you become more familiar with the exercise this can be increased to five breaths. With regular practice you will notice your breath becoming longer and deeper as your lungs expand more completely. Breathe in what nourishes and replenishes you the most, and use the outgoing breath to breathe away what you don't want, and to relax deeply.

In chapter 14, Creative meditations and visualisation, the lovely practice called 'the ocean of abundance' joins deep yoga breathing with the visualisation.

Alternate Nostril Breathing: *Nadi Shodhana*

Alternate Nostril Breathing is one of the most important pranayama practices, almost always taught in yoga classes. It is highly recommended for the health of the mind and the emotions, and is an excellent preparation for meditation because it quietens the mind and very quickly establishes stillness in the body.

The word *nadi* refers to the 72,000 channels for carrying energy from the spiritual body to the physical body. *Shodhana* means 'to purify or cleanse'.

By practising *nadi shodhana*, our energy channels—both physical and spiritual—are cleansed and purified.

In yoga philosophy, the left nostril is related to the *ida nadi* and the right nostril to the *pingala nadi*. The breath in the left nostril is cool and corresponds to the moon, and is known as *chandra nadi* (*chandra* means 'moon'). The breath in the left nostril corresponds to the right side of the brain, the feminine aspect and the creative, dreamy side. The breath in the right nostril is considered hot like the sun, and is known as *surya nadi* (*surya* means

> **Note:** If one nostril is blocked this simple procedure can help free the air flow enough to continue with the exercise. For the left nostril make a tight fist with the left hand and place it under the right armpit, while breathing through the left nostril. This will often encourage the breath to flow more easily. Reverse these instructions for the right nostril. The Breath Balancing posture (page 94) gives a similar result.

'sun') and corresponds to the left side of your brain, the masculine aspect and the analytical, practical part. The breathing exercises are one of the many ways of balancing and 'recharging' the nadis and the pranic body.

The benefits of Alternate Nostril Breathing are threefold. From a physical perspective, it helps balance the left and right sides of your brain as the breath flows evenly through both nostrils. It is an excellent practice for the respiratory system, toning and strengthening the lungs and airways. Oxygen is more efficiently taken in and carbon dioxide and toxins more efficiently removed. This breathing exercise greatly benefits those who are asthmatic or tend to breathe 'shallowly' or through the mouth, and sinus congestion is removed as the breath is encouraged to flow equally in and out of the nostrils.

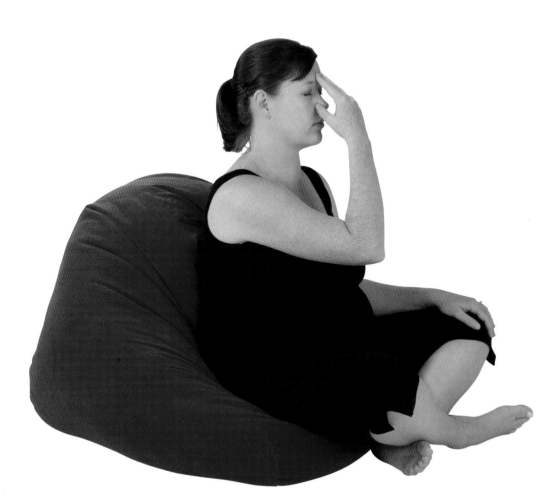

Secondly, this is an 'active' breathing exercise, as your awareness and concentration are focused on controlling the even flow of the breath. This helps to prevent your mind from wandering and enables your awareness to come more into the present moment. Mental and emotional stability are established and the physical action induces tranquillity and an overall sense of balance.

The third benefit is that *nadi shodhana* helps to purify the body and mind, creates an overall feeling that is calm and harmonious and the right 'atmosphere' in your mind for meditation.

Variation 1

1. Sit in a comfortable position with your spine straight and your body relaxed. Using your right hand, place your thumb beside your right nostril, your first two fingers between your eyebrows, and your ring finger beside your left nostril.
2. Block your right nostril with your thumb, and breathe slowly and evenly in and out of your left nostril,

Note: Sometimes you might find it too difficult to breathe through just one nostril. You can breathe in through one nostril and out through both nostrils or through the mouth until you feel comfortable with breathing out through one nostril.

three times. The breath is not meant to be deep for this exercise, just a little deeper than a resting breath and something you are completely comfortable with.

3. Change fingers, blocking your left nostril with your ring finger, and breathe three times in and out of your right nostril. If you are quite comfortable with this number, you can continue and repeat up to seven breaths through each nostril. Always do the same number of breaths on each side and always begin with the left nostril.

This breathing is meant to be slow, even and fluid and there should never be any discomfort, shortness of breath or difficulty. Practice for at least two weeks or until you become confident and relaxed with it, then advance to variation 2.

Variation 2

1. Begin with your hand in the same position as for variation 1.
2. With your right nostril blocked, breathe in though your left nostril.
3. Change fingers by releasing your right nostril, block your left nostril and breathe out through your right nostril.
4. Breathe in through your right nostril, change fingers and breathe out through your left nostril. Explained more simply, breathe in through your left nostril, out through your right, in through your right and out through

your left. This completes one round of the Alternate Nostril Breath.

5. Repeat this four more times to complete five rounds altogether. Try to breathe in and out evenly at all times. Do not hold your breath, allow yourself to become breathless or alter the pattern in any way. When you are competent with this technique the breath can be lengthened slightly.

The Cooling Breath:
Sheetali Pranayama

Many women in labour have successfully used the Cooling Breath, inhaling through the mouth, especially when used in between the contractions to help them remain centred and calm and restore lost energy. Other women have told of how it helped take their minds away from being fearful or anxious and stay focused on the present moment, enabling them to remain relaxed. It is a simple exercise involving very little effort other than feeling the coolness of your breath over your tongue as you breathe in.

It becomes an even more powerful technique when specific visualisations or images are used in conjunction. For example, before you begin to practise, bring to mind what your needs are at that moment, what will nourish and replenish your energies the most. Maybe you are feeling drained and fatigued during pregnancy, or you feel exhausted because labour has been long and difficult and it is energy you are needing. At another time you might feel a need to fill yourself with light, peace and calmness. You might like to visualise a specific colour that expresses these feelings and all these nourishing, positive qualities can be drawn in with the breath. These are all positive attributes of conscious breathing.

Another useful technique is to imagine your own special place in nature somewhere that makes you feel quiet and calm, confident and strong. This might be a familiar place or somewhere you have never been to, but just the thought of this place has a calming effect on you. Imagine these powerful yet gentle energies being drawn into your body, your mind and your spirit with each breath. This works with all the breathing exercises but especially with the Cooling Breath.

Sheetali pranayama cools your body and has a stabilising effect on your blood pressure, making it a valuable choice if your blood pressure is high or low. It is also said to be one of the most efficient ways of directing prana throughout your body or to specific parts of your body. With regular practice the blood becomes purified and your body will feel still and relaxed.

There are two variations of the Cooling Breath, one with your tongue relaxed in your mouth and the other with your tongue curled. Some people are genetically unable to curl their tongue and will find the second variation impossible.

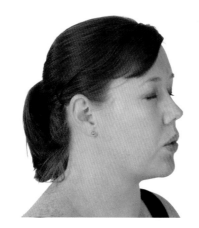

1. With your mouth in the shape of an O, as if you are going to whistle, breathe in slowly while feeling the cool stream of air over your tongue.
2. Close your mouth and breathe out through your nose. You can breathe at your regular breathing pace, up to nine times, or with slower, deeper breathing, maybe three or four times. Sometimes the Cooling Breath will make you thirsty. If you plan to use this technique during labour, sipping a little water every so often will help prevent dryness.

If you can curl your tongue, open your mouth, curl your tongue and breathe in feeling the air channelled through the tunnel shape. Close your mouth and breathe out through your nose.

The Hissing Breath:
Sheetkari Pranayama
The Hissing Breath is similar in procedure and benefits to the Cooling Breath. The only difference is the position of your mouth and tongue.
1. With your teeth a little apart and your lips slightly open, breathe in slowly and steadily.
2. Close your mouth and breathe out through your nose. You can breathe at your regular breathing pace, up to nine times, or with slower, deeper breathing, maybe three or four times.

This exercise is very good if you are feeling anxious or restless, making it especially relevant for the control of panic attacks. This exercise slows the incoming breath slightly and encourages you to control the flow of the breath better and to breathe more efficiently.

The Humming Breath:
Bhramari Pranayama
The word *bhramari* means 'large black bee', and when this exercise is done correctly the sound you make is similar to that of a bee. Some women find it a little difficult initially to produce a continuous, even humming sound with the exhalation, but with practice most women thoroughly enjoy it and often use it during childbirth and after the birth too.

Dr Wayne Dyer speaks at length about sound and its healing potential in his book *Manifest Your Destiny*—sounds 'are

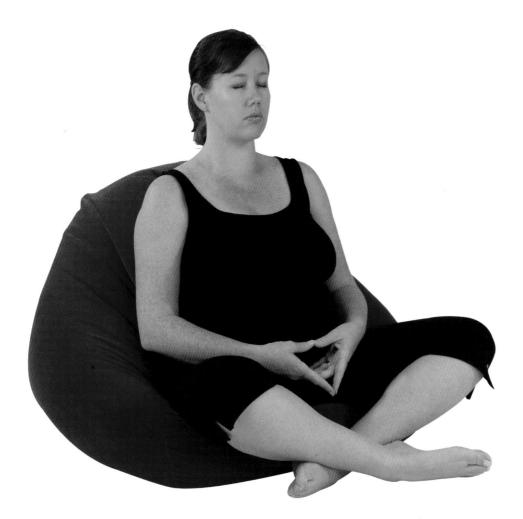

this sound is healing, the rejuvenating effects are often quite remarkable. As you hum, imagine the healthy cells in your body being enlivened and glowing with vitality, and any 'off colour' cells being either restored to health or eliminated. As you breathe in affirm the feelings that will nourish you and your baby the most and know that these thoughts are carried with the sound and vibration.

Many women have told me how their babies respond positively to humming after the birth. I think their babies remember the beautiful sound their mothers made when they were safe in the womb and the feelings it gave her and them too. Some women believe the humming breath helps to release natural endorphins during labour and for this reason it is valuable to consider during childbirth.

Kylie Lawless, mother of Tayla, says of the humming:

a powerful healing energy. Every sound is a vibration made of waves oscillating at a particular frequency … Sound has healing properties when it is harmonious and soothing' (page 113). He also mentions that women of ancient times apparently used the beautiful sound of *om* while birthing their babies (page 114).

The word *om* is well known in yoga and in many other spiritual sources. It is often said to represent the sound of the universe or the sound of God. The Humming Breath can be likened to the 'm' sound of *om*.

The primary importance of the humming breath is that the sound you make is your own unique healing sound, one that resonates with balance and wellbeing on all levels—the humming breath has a powerful healing influence on your whole being. When you hum your physical body benefits, the mind and emotions are calmed and your baby is bathed in this beautiful sound and healing vibrations. I'm sure your soul rejoices too. When you hum every cell in your body receives a beautiful healing vibration, like a soft massage and because you know

It's hard to put into words just how beneficial the humming was to my state of mind during pregnancy and now at home with my baby girl. I had never hummed before I became pregnant and now I use it often to help me relax and be still. Before I learned the breathing exercises I found it very difficult to slow my mind and to meditate as I always had a million thoughts running through my head, but when I discovered humming and how to focus my mind I was able to just be in the present moment. Humming made me feel calm, confident and relaxed and allowed me to concentrate on my breathing much more easily. I used it during labour and found it very helpful then, while now I use it to calm my daughter who responds to it almost immediately.

Lynn, another of my students, had been coming to yoga since the twelfth week of her pregnancy. When she was introduced to the Humming Breath she liked it immediately. During labour she used this exercise along with her birth support people, and found she was able to breathe down into her body, humming louder the more intense the contractions became. Listening to her own sound through each contraction enabled her to create the concentration and balance she most needed.

The Humming Breath helps initiate balance throughout your whole body and mind because of the soothing vibrations the sound creates. Even if you are still able to think while you hum—as some people are—when this technique is practised consistently, your mind gradually becomes quieter and more centred. The Humming Breath is very soothing for the nervous system and helps you to turn your awareness inwards, to be in touch with your 'inner being' and your baby. It is highly recommended for those times when you feel unsettled, anxious or angry, and it is particularly good for the relief of insomnia and extreme restlessness. It's worth remembering that people don't usually hum when they are angry or depressed.

When you hum continuously for three or four minutes, the silence that is experienced afterwards is one of pure peace and tranquillity. You might like to try this on a beach or in a quiet forest, humming for a while and then listening to the sounds all around you. Sometimes in my yoga classes we do a sound meditation where I ask the class to hum or chant *om* continuously, not counting the breaths so they are free to focus purely on the sound and the vibration. When they stop the room is filled with a beautiful stillness and the silence is transcendent, an atmosphere of serenity and wonderful calm. The women are as one with the healing sound and with the silence, and their babies feel it deep in their wombs. This is a beautiful way for women to nourish each other and their babies in the womb.

Everyone has a unique humming sound that resonates with perfect harmony for that person. Some people hum deep and long, while others will hum a little higher. When you are breathing slowly and deeply with your full awareness on maintaining a long gentle humming sound, you become one with *nada*, the psychic sound. Your thoughts, feelings and physical body become the continuous movement of sound, within you and all around you.

If you do this regularly during pregnancy, your baby will recognise your humming sound after the birth. This is especially good to do during breast feeding to relax you both, or afterwards as a lovely way to just be there together. Humming softly is a gentle way to comfort your baby if she has had a fright or is distressed in

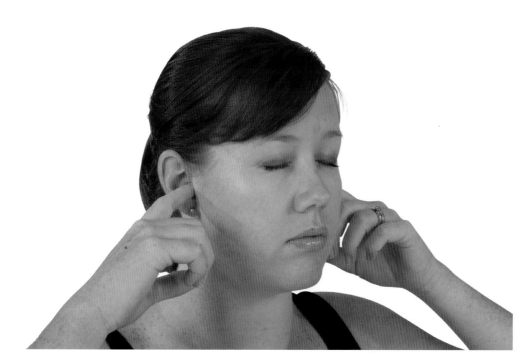

some way, or to calm a fretting and restless baby. A new mum told me she hummed when her baby was having a blood test and she said it definitely soothed her baby, and no doubt her too. For the singers among you, the Humming Breath is also recommended for improving your voice and strengthening your throat.

1. Sit in a comfortable position with your spine straight and your eyes lightly closed. The humming breath can be practised with your ears blocked or unblocked.

2. Breathe in and out through your nose, while making a humming sound as you exhale. Concentrate on the humming sound which will be quite loud inside your head when your ears are blocked.

3. Continue for nine breaths, or continuously where you are simply one with the breath, the sound and healing vibrations. Humming can also be practised three or four times with full complete breaths.

It is possible to hum with your jaw relaxed and your mouth a little open by pressing the back of your tongue against the soft palate. This is relevant for childbirth because of the association between your mouth and jaw being soft and open and the corresponding feelings in the cervix and perineum. This awareness encourages you to be open and relaxed to birthing your baby.

The Throat Breath, Breath of Tranquillity or Ujjayi Breath:
Ujjayi Pranayama

Ujjayi means 'psyche' or 'soul'. This gentle breathing exercise leads the practitioner into the more subtle, spiritual aspects of the self, to the soul. The Ujjayi Breath is the most valuable yoga breathing technique you will learn as a way to bring a deep sense of peace to the mind and present moment awareness. Its value as a life skill is unsurpassed. The Ujjayi Breath is especially beneficial as a birth preparation and is the breathing used more than any other during childbirth. It is also known as the Throat Breath because of the sensation felt at the back of the throat, and as the Breath of Tranquillity because of the soothing, relaxing effect it has on the mind and emotions.

It can be used simply as a breathing exercise with the soft natural breath, or with slow, deeper breathing. It is also excellent for concentration and contemplation, and done with that purpose in mind leads to deep meditative states.

Ujjayi breathing is a meditation within itself because it draws the awareness into a silent place, deep within our minds that is there beyond our thoughts. This enables us to realise the true nature of the mind—which is clear and luminous and where complete stillness is ever present. When ujjayi breathing is understood, we experience a feeling of complete oneness and peace with the self, as if time does not exist and there are no boundaries or limitations—as if we have stepped into eternity. When it is practised for longer periods, as in deep meditation, we move beyond the limitations of our minds to the vast eternal space known in yoga as *chitta kash*—the space of the conscious, subconscious and unconscious mind.

Used as a meditation the breath slows down to where it is barely felt in the body. The mind becomes one with the breathing, the movement of the breath, the sound of ujjayi and the soft sensation at the back of the throat. It is a complete meditation within itself. Many great teachers have referred to the mind as being like the sky, where in its purest form the mind is as clear and empty as a mid day sky. The clouds that move through the sky are only on the surface, and beyond them this vast, peaceful space is always present. In a similar way the clouds can represent our thoughts. Once we detach from the thoughts on the surface of the mind and simply become witness to them, we can access the mind as a peaceful space deep within us, just beyond thought. Close your eyes for a moment and bring your attention to the eyebrow centre, to the space of the conscious mind and watch the movement of your thoughts as they move in and out of the mind. When one thought ends and before another one begins there is a gap, a void, experienced as absolute stillness and peace. Now imagine what it is like beyond your thoughts—extend your awareness out through that space to sense a feeling of silence and incredible stillness. It's like looking into the sky and knowing it has no beginning or end. When time is spent doing ujjayi pranayama it is possible to rest in this space just for a moment, after you breathe in and before you breathe out.

Many of us search for external paths through which to bring quietness and calmness into our lives. But if we turn our awareness inwards, to contemplate, mindful, to be present, we will find the peace we seek outside ourselves is already there within our own minds. To meditate. Ujjayi breathing will help us access the more gentle aspects of the mind, especially when it is used for the purpose of meditation.

The throat breathing is always meant to be very gentle, but sometimes people are inclined to try too hard at first. If you strain and force your breath you will find the exercise difficult. The sensation at the back of the throat has been described as similar to breathing through a hole at the back of your throat. The sound is likened to a soft snore, like a sleeping baby's breathing or the sound you hear when you hold a seashell to your ear. (To a *Star Wars* fans it sounds like Darth Vader breathing.) When it is done correctly you will hear this soft sound and feel a very slight constriction at the back of your throat as you breathe in and out.

This exercise helps lower blood pressure because of its relaxing and calming nature. It can be done lying down making it a valuable technique if you wake at night and cannot go back to sleep, spending some time following ujjayi breathing will often put you back to sleep very quickly. It is also a perfect practice for those new to meditation, as your concentration can be focused on the movement of the breath, the sound of your breath and the sensation in your throat. The Ujjayi Breath has a threefold point of awareness that brings you to a oneness with the self. The more time spent practising this technique the slower and softer you will breathe, where you become one with the breath, in meditation with it.

Not all women enjoy practising this in the traditional way so I have incorporated a few modifications that make this valuable technique more available. As an alternative to using it for the whole breath, breathe in with the resting breath and out with ujjayi, or breathe in with ujjayi technique, and breathe out normally either through the nose or the mouth. This is an especially potent way to relax and release tension, as the practice itself is about relaxing, and breathing out through the mouth is always associated with release of tension and relaxation. This variation is of particular relevance for childbirth.

As explained for humming, ujjayi can be done with the mouth a little open and the tongue blocking the back of the throat.

During labour, ujjayi breathing can create a feeling of calmness in as few as three or four conscious breaths, and is ideal when resting between contractions. If you are interested in using self-hypnosis during labour, this technique is the best way of taking yourself into a deeply relaxed hypnotic space, and keeping you there longer. If you find yourself slipping out of relaxation or hypnosis, ujjayi breathing will take you back faster than anything else.

One of my clients, a speech therapist, said this technique put a slight pressure on the cranial nerves at the back of the throat and was therefore relaxing to the brain and the nervous system. The value of ujjayi breathing is truly extraordinary and in many ways it is the most valuable of all pranayama exercises.

1. Begin by sitting with your spine straight, your body relaxed and your eyes lightly closed. Place your hands in one of the mudras (chapter 9) or rest them on your abdomen. Concentrate for a moment on feeling the light sensation of the breath in the front of your nostrils.
2. Continue to breathe in and out through your nose, but now direct your breath towards the back of your nostrils, to the back of your throat and tongue.

If this is difficult to do, concentrate on where your breath is felt in your nostrils, then move your concentration away, as if bypassing them, until you feel as if you are breathing at your throat. When you do this correctly, you will feel a slight tightening sensation at the back of your throat and you will be able to hear a soft sound.

3. Continue on in this manner for as long as desired with your whole attention on your breathing. You will notice your breath becoming longer and deeper without having to make a conscious effort. It can be done with a quiet resting breath and included with deep yogic breathing and the deep cleansing breaths.

If you are unsure whether you are doing this correctly, block your ears and count five natural breaths and then five throat breaths. This way you will more easily hear the difference.

The Cleansing Breath

This is not a traditional yoga exercise but is recommended for its many benefits. It is done with the resting breath or in the same way as the Deep Yoga Breathing (page 98), the only difference being that the exhalation is through your mouth instead of your nose.

The Cleansing Breath has a powerful influence when your attention is not only on your breathing but includes the concept of blowing away any discomfort in your body, unwanted thoughts or confusion in your mind, and associated limiting emotions. Bring your attention to the tight or tense parts of your body, unwanted thoughts or uncomfortable feelings, and imagine you're blowing them away as you breathe out strongly through your mouth. In this way your breath and your conscious awareness are acting to cleanse your body and mind.

This is a powerful technique that is often used during labour either with the full breath, or with a softer natural breath where it can be done continuously. As mentioned for the Humming Breath and the Ujjayi Breath, keep in mind the association between the mouth being open and the lips being soft, and the pelvic floor muscles, the perineum and the cervix being soft, relaxed and open to birth your baby.

Breathe in deeply and slowly through your nose, then breathe out strongly and completely through your mouth as if you are blowing something away. This clears carbon dioxide from your lungs and encourages your body to relax deeply. Keep your attention on your breathing and on blowing unwanted thoughts, confusion or negative emotions out and away from your mind and tensions away from your body.

Repeat this three or four times if you are breathing deeply, or as often as you wish with when using the natural breath.

CHAPTER 12

MEDITATION

When the time came to write about meditation I found it an all-encompassing task. Endeavouring to explain the feeling experienced during meditation was challenging, indeed awesome. This is because meditation is in many ways beyond words, it is intangible, about feeling rather than form, the experience of pure simplicity in the truest sense. It is the art of being still. I practise meditation as part of my daily life and teach it regularly, but when it came to putting it in an easy to understand format this very simplicity became a stumbling block.

Until you make the effort to really take notice of what is going on in your mind, you are generally unaware that it is filled with a continuous stream of thoughts that move in and out without

any intent on your part. When you stop and observe what the mind focuses on, it is quite astounding—thoughts with no connection to each other that seem to come from nowhere and often with no relevance to the here and now—and all happening unconsciously. On average you will think over 100,000 thoughts every day! So it is not surprising that meditation is often very difficult when first attempted. Discipline and practice are required to make some peace with all this activity and to come a little closer to taming the wanderings of your mind even slightly. But in time you will begin to realise the many benefits attributed to meditation and that it is a precious gift you can give yourself. Meditation provides quiet time with yourself to bring the mind back home and be at peace with that.

Meditation comes from simply observing your thoughts. It is a gentle progression from being conscious that

you are thinking—that is, to stop for a moment and witness your thoughts—to being unattached, and mindful of your thoughts as they appear and disappear. In this unattached state you will be less caught up and distracted and just watch them, in the same way as you watch people walking past you—they are there and you are watching, nothing more. This leads to contemplation, where you are better able to relax and eventually become more still, and finally to a firm yet calm concentration on simply being the one who is watching, completely uninvolved and unaffected by the nature of your thoughts. It is not a matter of having no thoughts in your mind at all, rather a matter of distancing yourself from them.

Meditation is a state of restful alertness. Thoughts begin to lose form and definition, they start to dissolve a little until they are simply there, without being a distraction. Eventually there will be a gap, a space between one thought and the next, where you will experience a moment of stillness and absolute calm. When you come to this feeling, even if only briefly, it is transcendently beautiful. To rest in the quiet of your own mind and discover inner peace is very precious. Meditation evolves out of that ever-increasing calmness. It is learning how to tame the mind, to watch the constant flow of thoughts more passively so you become the witness to yourself thinking and to the crystal-clear yet transient domain of no thought. In meditation you bring the mind back to itself—like a dog on a very long lead racing off after anything and everything, with no direction and purpose, you gather the lead back to a more manageable length to tame the dog and keep it steady. It is the same in meditation—in time you become less distracted and steady and alert enough to concentrate on what you choose to, not on what the mind randomly decides to be consumed by. When you are meditating you focus with purpose and intention in the most peaceful way, which encourages a more relaxed, pleasant and easy mind state.

The gift of learning to meditate is the greatest gift you can give yourself in this life. For it is only through meditation that you can undertake the journey to discover your true nature, and so find the stability and confidence you will need to live and die, well.
Sogyal Rinpoche, *Meditation*

Meditation is an ephemeral expression of the mind and because of this it is maybe better understood by other terms. Concentration. Contemplation. Mindfulness. Inner stillness. One-pointed awareness. Inner reflection. In principle they are all the same and all eventually lead to the same place—a state of pure awareness. So how does one really explain what meditation is or accurately capture the essence of it in words? It is as simple as watching the wind moving gently in the trees and being one with that, yet as complex as contemplating the true nature of the mind and what life is all about. There are many books dedicated to this fascinating subject explaining the origins, the different teachings and various techniques, and how best to incorporate

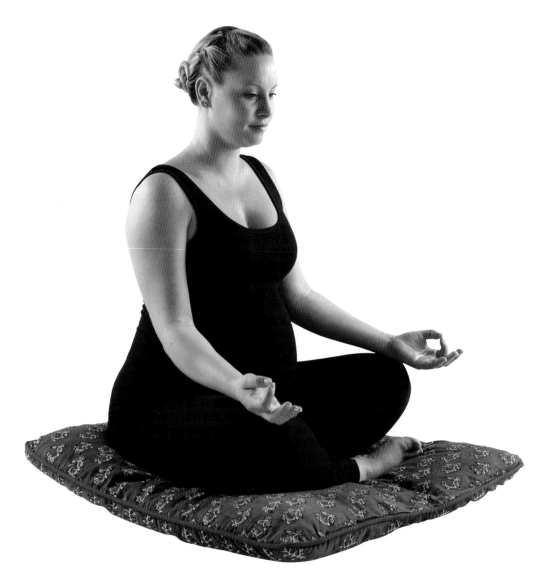

them into daily life, as well as the unlimited benefits it has for the mind and the body. I don't intend to go into such thorough detail here but instead keep it clear and simple. That is what meditation is in its purest form—clear and simple.

There are many different forms of meditation and many ways to approach it. What you choose to do is very personal, just as inner reflection and time spent alone with yourself are private concerns. No matter which path is best for you, all will eventually lead you to the same place, where you come to view and realise the world within yourself, in your mind—and find true contentment in time alone. To be at peace with yourself. Meditation can be felt as if you are finally coming home to yourself, to rest with your own spirit. In his book *Meditation*, the renowned Tibetan Lama Sogyal Rinpoche says, 'Meditation … is bringing the mind home.'

Some people come to meditation assuming the mind should be free of all thoughts. The mind, however, is rarely completely clear. There is always going to be a constant flow of thoughts, sometimes more invasive than at other times, as well as moments where there is space beyond or between them, and it is through the practice of meditation that you will come to enjoy precious, conscious moments in a more restful mind space. Thoughts are continually drifting in and out of your mind in the same way that clouds drift through the space of the sky.

Imagine being in a plane and all you can see outside are clouds. As the plane ascends it moves through the clouds, to eventually fly above them into an endless space where you view them unattached and from a distance. In the same way, when you meditate you move apart from your thoughts, you distance yourself, to experience the eternally still and peaceful sky-like nature of your mind, always there just beyond your thoughts. Another way to view this is to imagine a pond of still, clear water in which you can see fish swimming by. A crab disturbs the mud at the bottom of the pond, the water becomes cloudy and turbulent, and the fish are no longer visible. In the same way confusion and unsettled thoughts disturb the clarity and steadiness in your mind, so you are not able to think clearly and be present, your decisions are clouded. In time, however, the mud settles, the water clears and the fish become visible again. When you are absorbed in thoughts your mind is distracted from its clear and true nature, but when thoughts can be observed rather than attached to your mind becomes clear and still.

To gain the most from meditation you need to focus on the process of meditating rather than grasping for a profound experience. Simply appreciate the process of concentration and contemplation and the atmosphere this creates in your mind. When there is an understanding of meditation—where you are the observer and the witness to your whole self—all other yoga practices and techniques are enhanced tenfold. Whenever you are practising a yoga posture with a clear mind held firmly in the present moment, you are more fully in touch with how your body is feeling and the rhythm of your breathing. This prevents mental distraction, physical over-extension and straining, and your yoga postures become the whole practice—they are meditation in motion. Meditation and concentration can be there when you are doing your postures; mindfulness and inner reflection when you are practising pranayama; contemplation and present moment awareness when you are relaxing, working, driving the car or watching a film. Every moment of every day is an opportunity to be consciously here, now, in the present moment—in other words, in meditation with life.

Knowing how to meditate and observe yourself so you are truly living in the now makes each moment one to remember and enables you to live your life with gratitude and conscious awareness. This is a point worth considering as no one knows when their last moment will come. Being conscious of this very moment, even now as you read these words, as if it were your last, will hopefully be enough to encourage you to reflect on yourself, your life and our world, moment to moment and simply be more awake to each day.

All aspects of yoga are important. But without knowing how to be still and at peace with yourself, the other practices have far less impact and yoga's true value will not be appreciated and enjoyed. Time spent in quiet contemplation during pregnancy is nourishing and replenishing on every level of your being. Inner reflection is a special time to honour this brief and transformational time, to reflect on that and the undeniable miracle that is happening within you, and provides the opportunity and space in the business of daily life to be there with your baby.

Whenever I speak to women after a birth I ask which aspects of yoga helped the most. The predominant answer is the ability to concentrate and focus their attention on their breathing and on what is happening in their body—to stay present with the process of birth. Familiarity with meditation, mindfulness and present moment awareness enables women to breathe with complete awareness and stay centred and relaxed even during the more intense moments of labour, often without feeling dazed, confused or distracted by chaotic moments. They were able to manage the extremes of labour often better than they ever envisaged was possible for them. This is what conscious birthing is all about.

When you are not overwhelmed by a difficult situation, your calmness affects others around you in the same way. A number of women have told me how valuable they found meditation and breath awareness as they prepared for a caesarean delivery. Because these women were not distressed or anxious their birth support people were more relaxed too and in a better position to assist and comfort them. It's like a pebble being thrown in the middle of a pond, whose ripples spread unendingly to the edges of the water. If you, as the centre, can be calm and confident, it will positively affect all those who are there with you.

The meditation practices I outline here fall into two groups. The first group, in chapter 13, are traditional meditations from some of the great teachers of past and present which concentrate primarily on the mind, the senses, the breath and the body. The second group, in chapter 14, is made up of creative meditations and visualisation techniques which can be used in conjunction with the first group or on their own. Some will naturally appeal to you more than others and give you excellent results. I suggest spending time with all the techniques, as each one has its benefits. Eventually you might like to create your own meditations, combining your favourites from the two groups.

All these practices are uncomplicated and quite easy to learn from a book. There are many other outstanding traditional yoga meditation techniques, and inspiring Buddhist practices, but I feel these are best taught on a one-on-one basis from teacher to student. When meditation is kept straightforward and reasonably simple— where the technique is in many ways a part of your own nature—the results are always encouraging and more quickly recognised.

Concentration is the practice whereby one's ordinary, distracted, uncontrolled mind is developed to the point that it can remain powerfully, effortlessly, and one-pointedly on whatever object one chooses.
Dalai Lama, *The Way to Freedom*, page 174

Your particular personality type has a bearing on how easily you will slip into meditation. Some people realise a quieter atmosphere in their mind almost as soon as they begin to meditate and have no difficulty watching their thoughts and observing their feelings. These people are naturally very relaxed and find that meditation simply enhances their inborn nature and is really what they have always done when they need to take some time out. Other people find it almost impossible to relax and be still other than when asleep, where they are often as restless as they are in their waking hours. They have a lot going on mentally and find taming their minds very challenging—even counting their breaths to 10 without becoming distracted is impossible when they first attempt it. Sometimes it can take months to glimpse a brief moment of clarity and stillness—but with patience and perseverance they will be rewarded for their effort. If you are disciplined and determined to understand what meditation is and really want to appreciate the remarkable benefits it has to offer, I am confident that in time everyone is capable of success.

Some people find being alone with their

thoughts and feelings quite overwhelming and even unpleasant, and for a few it is just too confronting. When a person's life is in turmoil and extremely stressful they often fill their time with 'outer' activities, not allowing themselves the time to think about what is actually happening. In a situation where the mind is restless and over-stimulated it is better to practise the yoga breathing exercises rather than trying to meditate because it encourages quieter states of mind and eventually more manageable emotions. There was a stressful time in my life when meditation was just not an option and I relied heavily on pranayama and I was always amazed and grateful for its almost instant benefits. Pranayama has the potential to completely alter the atmosphere of the mind and ultimately establish much-needed calmness, so that meditation then becomes possible. The breathing is what you concentrate on and then becomes the meditation.

When someone is struggling with a difficult life issue or is new to meditation it is not uncommon for them to become unsettled or even emotional after a meditation, simply because it has been a long time since they have taken a few moments out for themselves, to just be, and discover that the quietness and stillness within themselves is both unfamiliar and extraordinary. For others, it means coming to a grinding halt where they have the opportunity to look at their lives in a more detached way and maybe find some positive solutions and alternatives to their usual way of doing things. I remember reading one of Dr Wayne Dyer's inspiring books in which he reminds us that we are human beings, not human doings—in other words it's okay to just be, we don't always have to be doing something.

Whatever your situation, always approach meditation slowly. If you become unsettled or anxious, open your eyes and only continue when you are ready. If you are having a lot of difficulty, rather than practicing on your own do so under the supervision of an experienced teacher. Sometimes your meditation practice will be fulfilling and deeply relaxing, at other times you will be easily distracted and not find the quietness and peace you so enjoy.

This is normal; meditation is like anything in life … sometimes when you bake your favourite cake using the same ingredients you always use, for some reason or another it doesn't taste as good as usual. It is important to emphasise that it happens occasionally to most of us, so don't be disheartened by a less pleasing result.

You have put in the effort and taken the time to be still, which helps bring about a feeling of wellbeing which is always replenishing and beneficial.

A life of only a single day spent in meditation, conjoined with wisdom, is better than living a hundred years unbalanced and confused.
> Dhammapada, in [first name] Choedak, [add *Book Title*], [omit date here 1996]

If meditation can be included easily into your daily routine or as often as possible, you will be more likely to include it as part of your life and health care program. Shorter sessions practised more often will keep you alert for the duration of the practice, rather than dozing off. You might find that 10 minutes is enough rather than aiming for a longer session in which you may be distracted by body or mind. Remember that meditation and mindfulness can be many other things than just sitting formally; it can be walking and being completely one with every step you take, it can be washing the dishes and feeling the warm soapy water on your hands and the smoothness of the plates. It can be in a conversation where you are mindful of your words, the tone of your voice and the way you are holding your body, and your breathing. Or sitting alone somewhere and watching the filtered sunlight on leaves or being moved by the beauty of a reflection on the water. Meditation can be listening to a breeze moving in the trees or just watching

waves rolling in and away from the shore. This is all mindfulness and concentration where your awareness is on less rather than more, focused and attentive. When you slow down enough to really observe your world and meditate on it, you appreciate it so much more and see beauty in the smallest things, in the unexpected treasures that nature is always offering. It can be everywhere and in every moment, during your pregnancy and after your baby is born.

Most pregnant women prefer to meditate sitting in a bean bag, their bodies as upright as possible. Others are comfortable in one of the traditional postures in chapter 10, Seated postures for pranayama and meditation. In a traditional seated pose you can sit with your buttocks on the floor or place one or two firm cushions under your tail bone. However, your seated position is less important than the meditation itself and it is essential to be as comfortable as possible so you are not distracted by your body. If you find these suggestions difficult, you might prefer sitting on a straight-backed chair with your legs uncrossed and your feet flat on the floor, or sitting on the floor leaning against the wall with your legs to the front, using cushions if need be.

Keep your spine as straight as possible so that your breathing continues to be smooth and even, and the muscles of your back and abdomen remain relaxed to allow vital energy to flow easily along your spinal column. Meditation is about the

mind and is always available to you and always valuable, whatever position you are in. This is especially relevant if you need to be in bed for part of your pregnancy or are unable to sit comfortably. If you need to lie down, make sure you are warm and comfortable, preferably on your side in the Flapping Fish posture (page 147).

I was taught to meditate with my eyes lightly closed and I suggest you practice this way too, although some teachings prefer the eyes slightly open. The choice is yours. Always do whatever gives you the best results, and this detail is less important than the actual practice.

Relax your arms from the shoulders and keep your elbows slightly bent. Rest your hands in one of the mudras, or place your hands on your abdomen to feel your baby in your womb.

Tilt your chin slightly downwards. Your lips are lightly touching and your teeth are a little apart so that your mouth and jaw are very relaxed. This softens the face and relaxes the muscles of your face, scalp, neck and upper body. Bring your attention to the position of your body. Your body needs to be as relaxed as possible for successful meditation, so pay particular attention to releasing tension before you begin and if need be change your position. When your body feels comfortable you will relax more easily and gain the most from your meditation practice.

Before you start your chosen practice, bring your awareness to your natural breath moving gently and evenly in and out of your body. I recommend 10 or 15 minutes of pranayama before you begin as this will help your body to relax and create a calmer more peaceful atmosphere in your mind. Through gentle breath awareness the environment of your mind becomes quieter, more still and centred. When you close your eyes to meditate you are alone with your thoughts and feelings and simply being the witness to the activity in your mind. From this quieter less distracted mind space your meditation can naturally evolve.

When you have finished your meditation, bring your attention to your natural breath once more. Gradually lengthen the depth of your breathing, each breath being a little deeper than the one before, feeling that each breath is bringing you more and more to present moment awareness. Notice the position of your body and your bean bag or cushions, the quietness in the room and then the sounds outside. Continue to deepen the breathing and spend as long as you need to come out of the meditation as gently as possible. Before you open your eyes take some slow, deep conscious breaths, drawing in all the nourishing qualities and feelings you want for the rest of your day.

When the time comes for your baby to be born, you will be able to use some of these exercises to help you stay calm and relaxed, and be present as you move through the birthing process. The more accustomed and skilled you become during pregnancy, the more easily they will come to mind during labour. Some women fear this knowledge will fly out the window during labour, but those who practise yoga and meditation consistently during their pregnancies always say they find themselves automatically doing their favourite techniques during labour, to their great benefit and relief. Even if these skills are used only briefly during childbirth, their benefits will still be felt then and afterwards as skills for the rest of your life.

Meditation is without doubt one of the greatest gifts you can give yourself and your baby during pregnancy, and for the rest of your life.

CHAPTER 13

TRADITIONAL MEDITATIONS

As you learn the traditional meditation skills outlined here you will see how they can be used on their own and together, and make the perfect place to begin any creative visualisation. They are invaluable as individual practices but also interact perfectly with each other, greatly enhancing what each has to offer. All eleven of these traditional meditations give a profound, deep meditation where the experience is unrestricted and totally free, especially when they are done in sequence, following on naturally from each other. For all meditation do at least 10 or 15 minutes of pranayama techniques beforehand to relax your body, settle your mind and establish the most appropriate atmosphere. Following the eleven specific practices are four examples of how they can be grouped together to create a balanced practice.

Breath Awareness

Breath Awareness is one of the purest and most consistently used meditative practices, found in most systems of meditation. It is the foundation of all meditation and mindfulness techniques. The breath is there with us every moment of our lives, it is our constant companion and a logical point of focus. Nothing external is needed, we have the breath within us to focus our attention on, any moment, any where—it is only a thought away. When we are exerting ourselves or stressed and anxious, the breath is more noticeable, often shorter and unsteady— and when we are calm and relaxed the resting breath is hardly noticeable at all.

Witnessing your breath quietly flowing in and out of your body as a form of meditation is uncomplicated and a most effective way of turning your awareness inwards. This enables you to observe the nature of your thoughts, the atmosphere they create in your mind and the natural rhythms of your body, and helps you to be totally present and clearly focused in each and every precious moment. (For more on this, see chapter 11, Breathing exercises.)

Three aspects of the breath can be followed for the purposes of this meditation:

- You can concentrate on the expansion and contraction of your abdomen as you breathe, the way your navel moves away from your body as you inhale and back into your body as you exhale, becoming completely absorbed in these movements.

- You can observe the movement of your chest as you breathe. Your chest expands as you inhale and contracts back into your body with each exhalation.

- The breath in your nostrils can be felt, with the subtle differences of a cooler breath as you breathe in and the less obvious, slightly warmer breath as you breathe out.

I suggest counting five breaths, with your awareness focused on the breath in your abdomen, then five breaths concentrating on the breath in your chest, followed by five more feeling the breath in your nostrils.

Each time you breathe in, feel you are drawing in all that is healing and balancing to you—the prana and life force available in each breath, and with it all the energies that are nourishing and replenishing. Breathing out, release all the unwanted feelings and thoughts that are preventing you from being relaxed and at peace. With each breath be mindful of the whole breathing process, observing yourself breathing in, and breathing out. Your breathing becomes the meditation, what you are concentrating on, with a one-pointed, steady awareness.

Breath awareness can also be done with ujjayi breathing where your attention is on the natural flow of your breath, the feeling in your throat and the soft sound of ujjayi. (For more detail see page 106.)

As you follow your breath it is natural for thoughts to come and go through the space of your mind. Rather than becoming attached to them, simply witness your thoughts and observe them in the same way as you witness your breathing, as you watch the movement of clouds passing across the open sky. Be mindful of yourself thinking and breathing. It's as if there are two parts to you, the one who is breathing and thinking, and the one who is watching you breathe and think.

When a thought arises, simply note that it has occurred, while at the same time remembering that it has come from nowhere, dwells nowhere, and goes nowhere, leaving no trace of its passage—just as a bird, in its course across the sky, leaves no mark of its flight. In this way, when thoughts arise, we

can liberate them into the absolute expanse. When thoughts do not arise, we should rest in the open simplicity of the natural state.
Dilgo Khyentse, *The Wish Fulfilling Jewel,*
page 85

The more time spent in the internal space of the mind watching yourself breathe, the more conscious you will be of the present moment and of any thoughts that come and go. After some time you will notice there is a natural gap, a space, between one thought and the next, where the mind is momentarily free of thoughts, or suspended between one thought and the one that follows. The pause between thoughts is very peaceful and sometimes feels eternal and infinite, as if you have stopped for a moment to simply be in that precise transient moment; it is the epitome of stillness. When you can hold your full awareness in this space, even for a brief moment, you witness pure awareness, the experience of pure bliss. You are in *dhyana* or meditation, in the space *chitta kash.*

Counting Your Breaths

Watching your natural breath is a valuable practice, but the mind being what it is will naturally roam and be distracted by unwanted thoughts, and therefore it is quite normal to lose constant breath awareness. Counting your breaths is a useful way of controlling the wanderings of your mind and staying focused. This can be done with your natural breath or ujjayi breathing. For increased focus

include the Breath Balancing Pose as well so you more easily notice your breath at the centre of your chest. You can count any number of breaths you choose, as a suggestion between five and ten breaths, repeating that number for as long as you do the practice.

Counting backwards is also an excellent exercise for improving concentration and staying focused on your breathing. When you first do this you might lose count very easily, but in time you will be able to watch your breath and count from a high number without losing concentration.

An effective method of taking yourself into a deep relaxation or meditation is to count down from 10 to 1, each breath being one count. With each descending number and breath feel yourself consciously and physically going deeper and deeper into the quiet and peaceful place within yourself. This is a self-hypnosis technique and because your intention is to be relaxed, most often by the time you have reached the count of 1 you are feeling quite calm and settled. If you are not, repeat the process as often as you need to. Once you are relaxed you can continue to follow your breathing or move into another meditation or visualisation.

Some women gain the best results when they breathe in with their focus on abdominal breathing, and exhale through the mouth. This is effective because the outgoing breath is always associated with relaxation and release of tension, especially when the mouth is open. The abdominal area is referred to as the emotional centre of the body, and whatever strong emotions we are feeling are 'felt' in the solar plexus and the stomach. This form of breathing has many benefits attributed to it especially for overcoming anxiety and reducing stress. Ujjayi pranayama can replace the natural breath for this practice.

The Ujjayi Breath

The Ujjayi Breath, described in detail on page 106, can replace the Natural Breath as a point of focus during meditation. It is a meditation within itself because the sound of the breath, the sensation of the breath at the throat and the whole breathing process can be concentrated on.

Ujjayi breathing is perfect for meditation, being a complete practice within itself. I have seen people practising it move very deeply into a quiet and peaceful place within themselves. It provides the opportunity to be alone and at peace with yourself and to maintain a firm awareness of the present moment. This Breath of the Soul enables you to be the witness and the observer of yourself and your breathing, and to occasionally move beyond your thoughts to realise that infinite space of the mind, the *chitta kash*—and to hold your awareness in that extraordinary space. The longer the technique is done the slower you will breathe and the more centred and still you will become. In essence, you are as one with the Ujjayi Breath, in union with

it. Yoga means 'union' and 'to join', and through this subtle meditation you are embracing what yoga is. After a time you will be able to let go of breath awareness and just be there, quiet and at peace.

You might like to begin this practice by blocking your ears and simply listening to the sound of the Ujjayi Breath quietly moving at your throat. If you have ever been snorkelling or diving you will know what it's like to be in a still environment and have the sound of your breath as a constant companion. In a similar way, when you spend time listening to the Ujjayi Breath or the natural breath, your attention will be drawn inwards as all other sounds become less obvious.

Focus on your natural breath and the air in your nostrils, then move your attention to feeling the breath at the back of your throat and listen to the sound of your breathing. Your throat might feel more open or a little constricted when practising ujjayi breathing. If you are feeling restless or are easily distracted,

practise with your ears blocked. When you are ready, unblock your ears and continue, simply listening and feeling the effects of the practice, or counting the breaths to hold your attention more firmly in the present moment. If you can retain your breath easily and comfortably, a short breath retention (*kumbhaka*) can be done now, just a brief pause after you breathe in and before you breathe out—so you become one with the whole breath, with the three aspects of the breath. When the breath is held for a moment, you are holding your awareness in a still and silent space—there is no breath, no sound and no sensation. This is the same feeling you have when you notice the gap between your thoughts, the same expansive stillness, inner silence and absolute peace, to experience the purity that is meditation and mindfulness.

It is very helpful to include the Breath Balancing Pose with ujjayi breathing, and affirmations or a mantra can be brought in for a very steadying and often profound result.

Ujjayi breathing in all its variations is the practice used more than any other during labour, either with a soft breath or incorporated into deeper breathing. Nearly all the women I have taught have used this technique at some point, especially between contractions, as an effective way to focus, to stay calm and strong in themselves.

Opening and Closing Your Eyes

During meditation it is quite common for people to relax so deeply that they drift off to sleep. This can be due to fatigue or to a sense of 'letting go' and allowing themselves to really relax, but sometimes it is because the meditation is going on for too long, especially for people new to meditation. I have found if the eyes are opened and closed intermittently, falling asleep is less of a problem and the meditation can be maintained for longer.

To gain the most from this practice, when your eyes are open focus on something that is just in front of you

and a little lower than eye height. This will prevent you from being distracted. When your eyes are closed feel yourself resting in a quiet inner space—each time this is repeated you withdraw more deeply inward and the experience is further intensified. When you open your eyes, even though you are conscious of what you see around you, you are less distracted, and in time will maintain the same quiet feeling with your eyes open as you do when they are closed, and enjoy some time alone with yourself. This practice enables you to feel the quiet atmosphere of your mind more fully, sometimes even more so than simply meditating with your eyes closed or following your breathing. It is especially useful when you are feeling restless and not able to move into meditation as easily as usual. Combine this with counting your breaths, say five to ten breaths with your eyes open, then the same with your eyes closed.

I also recommend this be practised with the Breath Balancing pose or ujjayi breathing.

Body Awareness

It is important to remember that whatever you focus your attention on during meditation will probably increase. If you concentrate on being calm, the feeling of calmness will usually increase. But if you have your attention on how anxious you are, the feelings of anxiety will probably increase, which can sometimes escalate

to the point where you have less control over your behaviour and emotions. This is especially relevant to childbirth.

The more conscious you can become of how you are feeling—physically and emotionally—the better you will be able to handle difficult or challenging situations, especially when they take you completely by surprise. When you are more consciously aware of yourself and have learnt how to be the observer and the witness, you are more likely to know whether you are relaxed or stressed by the way you are feeling in your body, by the nature of your thoughts—and especially by the way you are breathing.

The next time you are relaxed, spend a few minutes simply observing yourself— aware of your body and how you are holding it, what you are thinking about, the sound of your voice and particularly how you are breathing. Likewise, if you find yourself in a difficult situation, watch and learn from what you do, how you feel in your body and how you react. Remember meditation and mindfulness can be in all aspects of daily life, not just in formal practice.

Although Body Awareness is a very simple exercise, it has many benefits and will help you to understand yourself more intimately. It is a significant life skill that will prove invaluable throughout your life.

The body awareness meditation can be done anywhere and at any time—all that is required is to stop and bring your attention to yourself. It can be used as a brief exercise for becoming centred and mindful, or as a prelude to other meditation practices. It can also be the whole meditation practice, where you reflect on all aspects of your body as you do in deep relaxation. Your focus can be held on your face, for example,

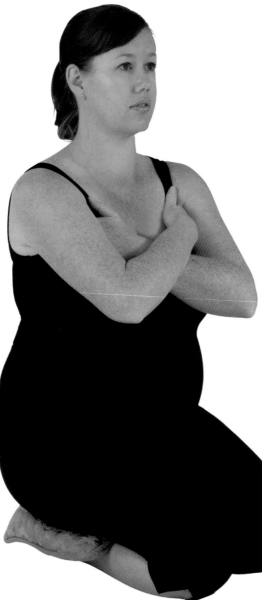

concentrating on the different features as well as your whole face and how soft it feels. You would then move your attention slowly to other parts of your body, observing them in the same unattached manner, but with full concentration.

Often it is observing the little things about ourselves that has the most impact. These simple observations means you are really embracing life as it happens, so that when something 'enormous' happens your awareness is finely tuned and you experience the moment more consciously.

Body Awareness brings you the opportunity to spend time contemplating your pregnancy and observing the changes in your body while honouring yourself in all your womanly beauty during this time. It is also a wonderful opportunity to spend time connecting with your baby, noticing the movements increasing and changing as she develops and grows to maturity.

Body Awareness is a valuable asset in labour as a way of 'bringing the mind back home'. It will hold your attention in the present moment and help you to remain calm, relaxed and centred as you progress through the contractions. In the case of needing a caesarean delivery, it will enable you to be as relaxed as possible while you prepare for the procedure. Body awareness is a simple and powerful mediation that is pure mindfulness in every way.

An excellent body awareness practice is to focus on your baby's movements in contrast to

the movements of your natural breath. This more difficult concentration exercise encourages the development of awareness. The difference between the two is quite subtle but this exercise clearly distinguishes one movement from the other. From there, you can then concentrate on the contrast between these movements and the feeling of complete stillness in other parts of your body. This is a valuable concentration practice, for when you move your attention slowly from movement to stillness, the distinction between the two gradually becomes more and more obvious.

From these movements now feel the contact points of your body with the floor and with your cushions, and where your body is in contact with itself—your hands resting on your abdomen, or in a mudra, or maybe your hair lightly touching your face. Feel very relaxed in your body as you continue—and again mindful of your breath gently moving in and out of your body.

Now feel you are so relaxed you start to feel heavy, and gradually becoming more so, where this heavy sensation becomes your complete point of focus. After a time reverse that awareness and feel your body is becoming light, and then lighter—so light that if feels like a feather floating on a breeze.

These are all aspects of Body Awareness and can be done so that one follows the other to progress into deep relaxation and meditation. Take as long as you need to move from one sensation to the next and then finally create the feeling of complete stillness in your whole body. The stillness you experience is quite extraordinary. When held as a meditation and in firm concentration, you begin to feel as if you are as still as a statue, like a rock. If your baby is sleeping your breath is the only movement you will feel in your body and because you are so relaxed, it is hardly moving at all. This now becomes a very profound and beautiful meditation. You are totally aware, mindful and present. You have finally detached from your breath and your body, to come to a place of complete calm, to be as one with your inner self, and at peace with that.

While holding that calm awareness begin a very slow, soft ujjayi breathing, watch how internalising it is, how long it takes you to breathe in and to breathe out. Your breath seems as if it is moving in slow motion, and when you do this for a length of time, it actually is when compared to regular breathing. You are totally conscious, very still and completely relaxed.

Breath and Pranic Body Meditation

This meditation is based on a traditional Kriya Yoga practice and follows on naturally from the Body Awareness and Ujjayi meditations. Although it could be considered advanced in nature it is also very easy to do. If you enjoyed the previous one, you will appreciate this

lovely meditation too. Pregnant women seem to move very deeply into their meditations, especially as they come closer to the time of birth, and many have enjoyed the almost transcendent experience that is felt from this practice. I have included it here because of the extraordinary feelings it gives to the physical body and the atmosphere it creates in the mind, one that is deeply relaxing and most peaceful.

When you have relaxed completely and feel as still as suggested in the previous meditation, gently move into soft ujjayi breathing again, where it is barely moving in your body. As you inhale feel not only the breath expanding in your chest and abdomen but as if your whole body is expanding as you breathe in, and contracting back again to its resting size and shape as you breathe out. As you continue to do this, each time you breathe in you seem to grow larger, or an aspect of you does, and as you breathe out you contract back again. This is prana moving in your body expanding with every breath—it feels like your physical body but it is your pranic body that is becoming twice as big and three times as big—and it continues to grow as much as you can imagine it to. Some women like to use colour or light to enhance their visualisation so that is what they see and feel as they follow the breath.

As you imagine you are expanding and contracting, you will actually feel as if your body is getting bigger, and the

question is whether it is just your firm concentration and your imagination or that you are really feeling your life force, the pranic body moving as well. Continue to do this, and then at some point when you are ready just let go of the breath and body awareness and simply be that pranic energy, colour or light—absolutely still, weightless, free, at peace. You might like to imagine you are looking at yourself sitting still and peaceful, see your face and the soft expression, see your whole body in its seated position, the shape of your abdomen and the breath moving very gently in and out of your body. Hold that awareness for as long as you wish and finally see yourself surrounded in a beautiful golden light and your baby in your womb with the same radiance glowing all around her.

The benefits from this, one of the most relaxing and deeply meditative of all practices, are many. This is an ideal place of mindfulness and contemplation from where to do your affirmations, to feel fully nourished, to be with your baby, to pray if you wish, to feel gratitude for your life and for the gift and grace of a new life within your body.

Sound Awareness

Listening to different sounds can be a valuable form of contemplation and meditation. The humming breath is an ideal sound for meditation, especially as you know the sound you make is your own unique healing sound, and one that your baby also hears deep in your womb. (Humming as a meditation is discussed more fully on page 103.) Sound meditation can also be practised through om and other forms of sacred chanting. Any of these can be done continuously, when they become powerful meditations within themselves. There is a traditional sound meditation called kirtan, comprised of mantras repeated continuously, set to the music of Indian instruments. Sound awareness might be done by simply listening to the different sounds of nature—a beautiful way to relax and turn your attention inwards, to focus on less rather than on more.

The sounds of nature are always changing and incredibly varied, and using them as a meditation practice is purifying and uplifting. Sitting in a forest or in a park on a windy day where the trees are making a wide range of sounds can be quite energising, as is listening to the surf pounding on the shore, or heavy rainfall. Then there are the softer sounds of nature which are more soothing and comforting to the senses, such as the gentle movements of a breeze in the trees, the sound of light rain, of a stream, or birds communicating with each other.

Once you are fully involved with listening and can concentrate on simply observing sound, it's amazing what you become aware of and the variety of sounds you will hear around you. Remember, in meditation whatever you focus your attention on usually increases. So, when

you really listen and hear what is around you, you will realise there is an unlimited variety of sounds in your world to be explored and enjoyed. Imagine using your mind like a radar system, where you listen to the closer sounds and the louder sounds, then to the quieter, softer sounds that are farther away in the distance.

Another practice is to listen to the sounds outside the room, and compare them to the sounds inside the room. This is a particularly valuable technique for being aware of the difference between the place where you are meditating, and the outside environment. In many ways it's comparable to present moment awareness—listening to the outer sounds is similar to the thoughts being on the external, and when you are consciously aware of the sounds inside the room or of your own breathing, your attention is directed more towards the internal environment. You are then less distracted, and more present.

As you master the art of conscious listening, you will be able to extend your awareness far beyond what is audible, to hear the silence that is beyond all sounds, to rest in a space that is clear and still. Then, as you bring your awareness back to what is around you, you will notice that the 'silence that is beyond the sounds' is also there around you, and eventually will be felt within you. The feeling is one of absolute calm, a gentle inner reflection and mindfulness. In many ways this is comparable to realising the infinite space

of your mind that is past the activity of your conscious mind, where you come to realise the true nature of your mind, that it is always still and peaceful.

If you can meditate in a very quiet place, you will more easily observe this silence and stillness, to a point where you immerse your whole awareness deeply into your self, to hear only the soft sound of your breath. When you become completely absorbed with hearing your gentle, natural breath, there is a perfect quiet within your body and your mind. You can then rest and be at peace with your self, with your soul.

In this way you will discover the similarities between the peace, stillness and silence you perceive beyond sounds, and that which you will discover deep within yourself. Ultimately, you bring the mind 'back home', to an atmosphere of complete calm.

Sense Withdrawal

This meditation is a variation on a very traditional practice and is easy to do with quite remarkable benefits. It is a combination of some of the other practices detailed here where the senses are gradually withdrawn from the outer senses to the inner space of the mind, to a place of stillness, peace and clear awareness. Commence with sound awareness and spend time listening to yourself humming and then to the sounds outside, those that are loud and those that are softer, and those that are further away in the distance. Spend as long as you need to be as one with external sounds. Then bring your attention to your body and your breath and feel your body and the movement of the breath. This can include awareness of your baby in your womb, and it is acceptable to complete the meditation there. Then to continue, be mindful of smell, concentrating and observing the sense of smell, and then taste. (Taste is discussed more fully in the Sultana Meditation on page 143.) From there draw your awareness to the space of the mind, beyond all the senses and movement in your body, to come to rest there, at peace with yourself. This can be done in a little as ten minutes or extend to half an hour or more. From this quiet inner calm, mindfulness, inner reflection and contemplation are possible. You are in meditation and will feel still and at peace.

Mantra Meditation

A mantra is a few words that are repeated continuously as a way to encourage the mind to stay focused and present. Mantras are different to affirmations, where you know the meaning of the words you are repeating—in a mantra the words are unknown to you, they may be Sanskrit, a Tibetan Buddhist phrase, or something given to you by your spiritual teacher. The purpose of a mantra is to not be attached to its meaning, but simply to repeat the words as you breathe and allow that process to centre your mind and hold you there in that moment.

Sometimes their meaning is relevant, but this is not essential. The belief is that if we don't know what the words mean we are less inclined to intellectualise about them and be distracted with meaning, and can therefore stay with a clear and present mind state more easily. This is suitable and appealing for some people and in many situations, for at other times the meaning your words carry will have great significance and often change the course of your mental activity. It is very personal decision, as both mantra and the use of affirmations in meditation are very worthwhile.

A mantra that is often used is to repeat the words *so hum* with the breathing. The word *so* is repeated in your mind as you inhale, and *hum* is repeated as you exhale. This can be done as a meditation on its own. It can also be used during your favourite visualisation, while your eyes are closed in the Candle Meditation, or simply as a way to steady your mind apart from formal practice. Repetition of a mantra is valuable during meditation if you become distracted by the activity of your mind and can't be detached from your passing thoughts, or if you become too analytical about your affirmations. Particularly when used together with ujjayi breathing, a mantra can be an effective way of moving deeper into relaxation and hypnosis, especially if you find yourself drifting out of that atmosphere.

In the last weeks of your pregnancy mantra can help you fall asleep again, if you are awake constantly due to pressure on your bladder or if your mind is overly active, or after the birth between night feeds to help you fall asleep. Some women have used this technique to their benefit during labour, between contractions to help them refocus and regather their mental energies, so their mind is steady and prepared for the next one. This is often done in conjunction with deep conscious breathing and ujjayi pranayama.

Begin by following your natural breath, if you wish counting your breaths to hold your awareness there initially. When you are ready begin repeating your chosen mantra. Some women prefer to repeat their mantra only as they breathe in, and just feel a soft relaxation settling in their body and mind as they breathe out. It really depends on the mantra and how it is best used, and importantly what you benefit the most from. There is no time limit on this meditation and mantra can really be done anywhere and at anytime. When you have been practising mantra meditation for some time, just allow it to gently cease, find yourself going beyond it and the breath, to simply rest in a quieter mindfulness where you can enjoy peace and contentment with yourself.

The Gaze: *Trataka*

The word *trataka* means 'to look' or 'to gaze'. This lovely practice helps to improve concentration because where the eyes are directed the mind and thoughts will follow. It is very simple to do and involves concentrating on a single stationary object, the purpose being that when the eyes are still and focused the mind is encouraged to do the same. The Gaze is one of the easiest and most beneficial meditation techniques, and ideal for those new to meditation, or when other practices do not give the benefits you are seeking. Its benefits are felt usually the first time you practise. *Trataka* very quickly brings tranquillity and calmness

to even the most over-active mind, and is therefore relaxing in a physical sense also.

You can choose any object you feel is easy to look at, but it needs to be something that won't create ideas and thoughts that will be distracting rather than centring. For example, you could use the face of a spiritual person, a religious symbol, a flower or a crystal, even a dot on the wall, as long as your focus remains on the one stationary object.

I often teach this technique to people who are stressed and in need of rest and relaxation, or who are unable to follow their breath because thoughts and worries flood their mind and prevent inner stillness. It is simple enough to do at home, which is important because it gives a positive sense of taking responsibility for your own health and wellbeing.

The Candle Meditation

In traditional yoga, the brightest point of a candle flame is often used for *trataka*. It is one of the easiest ways for people new to meditation to understand what it is and to experience its benefits. Very little effort is required other than to gaze at the brightest point of a still candle flame—it is easy, calming and quite mesmerising. This meditation has always been a favourite with pregnant women.

The candle meditation is one of the surest ways of establishing a quiet state of mind and learning how to focus, and can be enjoyed in a class situation and at home. It can be used in pre-labour at home to help you relax and stay calm before the more active part begins. Once you are in hospital, where it is not permitted to have open flames, you can keep the image of the flame in your mind to act as your visualisation and concentration point. If you are having your baby at home you might like to have lit candles to create a peaceful and warm ambience during labour.

For those who suffer from insomnia or are restless sleepers, this is an effective way of relaxing before going to bed, to induce a better night's sleep. A client of mine had been using sleeping pills for a number of years and decided to practise candle gazing every night for 20 minutes before going to bed. She found after only a few days that she no longer needed her sleeping pills.

Trataka will strengthen your eyes and gently stimulate your brain via the optic nerve, making it ideal in conjunction with other eye exercises. It can be practised on its own or before your other meditations and breathing exercises as a way to become quiet and relaxed.

For the best results, practise this meditation at night in a darkened room. If you practise during the day, make the room as dark as possible. You will also be less distracted if the background to the candle is a blank wall.

Sit in a comfortable position or in a bean bag and relax your body completely. Place a lighted candle at least an arm's length from your face at eye level. Make sure there is no breeze in the room so that the flame remains as still as possible. This

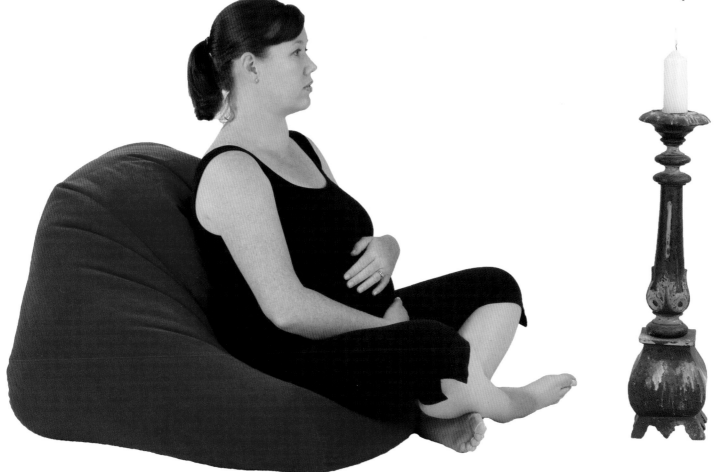

is important because the idea of *trataka* is to encourage the mind to become still—if the flame is moving even slightly, your mind will be inclined to move too. Rest your hands on your abdomen, or in one of the mudras. If you enjoy the Breath Balancing pose, use this to gain the benefits from both practices.

Close your eyes and bring your awareness to your body and the flow of your natural breath. Be aware of the nature of your thoughts and the atmosphere they are creating in your mind. Take some slow, deep, conscious breaths to establish deeper relaxation and peace of mind in readiness for meditation.

When you are ready, open your eyes and gaze at the brightest point of the flame. Blink if you need to and always close your eyes if your eyes begin to sting or water a little. Sometimes this happens when you first practise *trataka* or if your eyes are tired or strained.

After two or three minutes, close your eyes lightly. Keep them closed for a short time as you observe your thoughts and your natural breath. When you are ready open your eyes and gaze at the flame again. Repeat this procedure as often as desired. To maintain a firm concentration while your eyes are closed I suggest counting your breaths, either with your natural breath or with ujjayi breathing, or repeating a mantra. The longer you spend gazing at the flame, the more centred and at peace you will become. After some time you will notice an 'internal' image

of the flame at the 'eyebrow centre' or in the middle of your eyebrows, when *trataka* becomes an open and closed eye meditation. You can use this pure still light in the mind to meditate on, or you might like to do a more creative meditation. Imagine a soft radiant glow from the flame all around your body, either very close to you like a silhouette or much larger; this can create a feeling of safety and peace. Or you might like to have your womb filled with a beautiful luminous glow surrounding your baby with feelings of love. Both these images can be also seen as coloured light to benefit from the healing in colour.

The Candle Meditation is generally practised for 10 to 15 minutes, but this can be shortened or lengthened to suit. If you are uncomfortable in a seated position or feel you need to lie down, rest on your side in the Flapping Fish posture with cushions for comfort. The candle can be placed at eye height at whatever distance feels best. This is a lovely way to practise this meditation and also worthwhile if you want to just drift off to sleep—making sure, of course, that your candle is safe. Pregnant women really enjoy this meditation while relaxing in a warm bath perfumed with some of the essential oils for pregnancy (see page 152).

Four Meditation Practices

These traditional practices can be combined to form a balanced, deep meditation practice. I describe four

meditations here, but when you become familiar with them you can change them to better suit you. The way you put them together is very much a personal choice. There is no time frame—your meditation practice might be as short as 10 minutes, or longer than half an hour.

In time you might like to create a very personal practice incorporating a selection from the creative visualisations in chapter 14.

For any meditation sit in a comfortable position with your spine straight, your back relaxed and your hands in a mudra or resting on your abdomen. Spend between 10 and 15 minutes doing a selection of your breathing exercises to steady your mind.

Meditation 1

Begin with simple breath awareness, following the movement of your natural breath for a short time until you are centred and present. Repeat three slow, deep, conscious yoga breaths and, after a short pause, three deep cleansing breaths.

Continue watching your natural breath and include counting your breaths in sets of 5 to 10, repeating that as many times as you wish. Then focus with your awareness on the breath in your abdomen, counting your breaths there. Then move your attention to your breath in your chest, repeating the same number of breaths, and then with your awareness in the nostrils, again counting your breaths. Then count the same number of breaths with a soft cooling breath so your awareness is on the cool stream of air in your mouth. Then practise ujjayi breathing so that it becomes your meditation—your concentration is on the movement of your breath, the sensation in your throat and the soft sound of the breath. You are then one with the technique and your breathing. This can be done for as long as you wish and followed with a creative visualisation of your choice, or deep relaxation.

Meditation 2

Begin with the Candle Meditation. Place your candle flame at eye height and about arm's length, then close your eyes. Bring your awareness to your natural breath, either counting your breaths or maybe repeating your mantra or affirmations. When you are ready open your eyes and stare at the flame, after a time closing your eyes lightly. While your eyes are closed continue counting your breaths or continue with your affirmation, or just stay with a quiet breath awareness and the image of the flame inside your mind at the eyebrow centre. Repeat this process as many times as you wish, including ujjayi breathing when your eyes are closed for a deep result. You might then wish to include a visualisation based on the light from the flame, or another visualisation you enjoy.

Meditation 3

Begin with simple breath awareness, this time with your hands in the Breath Balancing pose to enhance your concentration. Focus on your breath at the centre of your chest, either counting your breaths or repeating your mantra or affirmation. When you are feeling calm and very relaxed, include ujjayi breathing and become one with it. Continue with this—the more relaxed you become the slower your breathing will be. You might like to spend some time with your eyes open, and then closed, counting an equal number of breaths, continuing for as long as you wish. When you finally keep your eyes closed just be in that moment, without mantra or affirmations, not counting your breaths, or even breath awareness … simply there, at peace with your inner world, with the wonderful, soft relaxation in your body and a deep stillness in your mind and your soul. The body awareness meditation can now be done and then the pranic body breathing practice. Continue with that and when you are ready include light or colour, completing the meditation by seeing yourself and your baby surrounded in a golden radiance. From this inner reflection spend some special moments with your baby, with thoughts of love and welcome.

Meditation 4

Begin by placing the hands across your chest in the Breath Balancing pose, either with the candle again or just following the movements of your natural breath at your chest. Proceed as suggested in the previous meditation and when you are ready include humming as well. This is especially valuable when the hands are across the chest because you will feel the movement of your breath deep in your chest as you inhale and the vibration of the humming as you breathe out. With your awareness solely on breathing in and humming as your breathe out, you will eventually find yourself in a beautiful rhythm with the breath, the sound and the vibration. There is no time limit on how long you practice the humming.

As you breathe in you might like to bring a loving thought to mind for your baby, or one to nourish yourself. Again, there is no time limit on how long you continue. When you decide to stop humming, imagine the vibrations there in your body and observe the softness of your breathing. Become absorbed in listening to the silence around you, be conscious of your inner calmness and know that your baby is resting in your womb in a gentle atmosphere of peace too. You might then like to take your awareness outside to hear all the sounds out there, the loud and the soft, those that are closer and those that are further away—then back to the silence in the room and finally to the sound of your natural breath. This can then evolve into the sense withdrawal meditation, where you can come to rest with your thoughts on your baby or in the clear space of your mind.

CHAPTER 14
CREATIVE MEDITATIONS AND VISUALISATION

The meditations in this chapter are creative visualisations that can be practised on their own, following on naturally from the traditional ones, or after the breathing exercises. This more peaceful aspect of yoga is what many pregnant women most enjoy. These meditations are about nourishing yourself as a pregnant woman and focusing on the importance of this special time. They include specific visualisations for enjoying quiet inner reflection with your baby in your womb. Many of them are favourite visualisations that women continue to request even when they come back to my yoga classes for subsequent pregnancies. In a way these meditations are their choice, their gift to you as you embrace your pregnancy and motherhood.

The first three meditations are most important as they focus on nourishing yourself during your pregnancy, your baby in your womb and the miracle of birth.

Honouring Yourself

This very special meditation is in many ways a summary of what this book is all about—honouring and nourishing yourself as a woman and a mother during the brief time of your pregnancy.

Your journey through pregnancy, when put into perspective against the whole of your life, is such a brief moment that it is often over before you have the opportunity to really become absorbed in all that has occurred. While you are pregnant and dealing with morning sickness, the loss of your waist, increased weight, fluid retention, fatigue, fluctuating emotions, headaches, backache, pubic pain, swollen feet, varicose veins, the occasional hot flush … and all the other things that can accompany a normal pregnancy, you can too easily miss the beauty of the changes taking place moment to moment. Or simply might not have the time to reflect on the absolute radiance that becomes you as you progress through your pregnancy. Women are often at their loveliest when they are with child.

It is important to stop for a moment and reflect on these rare moments—brief as they are—and allow yourself the luxury to be at peace with the miracle that is happening to you.

For many women the idea of becoming a mother is an awesome thought filled with varied emotions including wonder and joy as well as fear and anxiety. It also brings with it a completely different kind of love—a love you will recognise the moment your baby is born, or often earlier during your pregnancy.

Honouring yourself does not need to be a formal meditation, but just some time away from the usual activities of your day where you can be alone and at peace with your thoughts and feelings. Such private moments and inner reflection will help you to appreciate that your life will never really be the same once your baby is born—but it will be enriched beyond words. This is a completely new beginning in so many ways.

Meditation of this type will keep you more 'present' in your pregnancy and help you to hold the essence of what it really means to be a mother. Long after your child is born and takes those first magical steps into their own new world, is waving good-bye to you on the first day of school, is taller than you and leaves home—you will appreciate the time you spent in quiet reflection during your pregnancy. Through meditation you will forever hold those images and feelings in your heart and soul. When your child eventually achieves these milestones you will realise how quickly time has gone, and a little inner reflection, together with the special joy and wonder that women often feel when they look at their grown children, will somehow soften the sad feelings that linger just behind a smile, remembering a time that doesn't seem so long ago.

Remembering to take a few moments in you day to pause and simply be, will encourage a quieter, more peaceful state of mind, where you bring your mind back home to itself to contemplate, to meditate and be present—to be alone and at peace with yourself. When you put the world on hold for a moment and create the opportunity to really enjoy this brief time, it is always nourishing and replenishing. It provides the space for you to connect with your inherent feminine wisdom, your baby and the miracle of life.

Your Baby in Your Womb

This is a beautiful meditation where you spend time with your baby in quiet contemplation before the birth, and is where much of your focus will naturally be during pregnancy. It also holds within it the true meaning of conscious birthing—awareness of your pregnancy and reflection on your unborn baby. For many women this can be a very moving meditation where strong, nurturing emotions arise from deep within, feelings that are unique and familiar to all mothers about their children.

It is also an important practice if women find it difficult to actually connect with the baby growing and developing in their womb, or grasp that it is a real person. Visualising your baby in the womb enables you to imagine what she might look like and to spend some special moments with her before the birth. Even if you're not able to create a clear picture in your mind, by spending time thinking about your baby your instinctive maternal feelings will begin to flow and the remarkable union of mother and child will start to take place.

For some women, the idea of having conversations with this 'unknown' in their womb can be a little difficult, especially when you are only in the early weeks of pregnancy, but as your pregnancy progresses you will find it easier and look forward to these quiet times together.

This meditation is especially valuable if you were at first unaware of your pregnancy and feel you have missed out on the early months, or were just too unwell to think about your baby. Because the future can't be predicted, it is worth doing from early pregnancy, if it happens that your baby is born earlier than expected. The same applies if the labour was difficult and your energy was taken up with recovering your strength, or if circumstances following the birth prevented you from spending the early days together. Using this meditation, much of the 'getting to know you' and bonding will have occurred long before the birth, so that you feel connected to your baby no matter what happens before or after the birth.

Rest in a comfortable position and bring your attention to your natural breath, spending as long as you need to relax your body and quieten your mind. Place your hands on your abdomen to feel your pregnant belly and your baby in the womb.

Bring your awareness to your baby, feeling her moving as well as visualising her. When you think about your unborn baby it is your child's unique self and personality that you are connecting with as much as the physical form. Your baby is a new soul, a divine, precious and unique individual. Each new child is a blessing from God—like a spark of brilliant light that has entered your body for the duration of pregnancy. Imagine your baby inside your womb carries this 'light' of a new life—a light that emanates from within her body and fills your womb with a beautiful radiance. Hold this image in your mind and be there with your baby. Your baby will feel the love in your thoughts.

Now imagine your baby's delicate features, the shape of the head, the eyes and the eyebrows, the tiny nose and nostrils and other features of your baby's face. Visualise the curved shape of the back and the legs tucked up in the foetal position, the little toes and even the tiny toenails. See your baby's arms floating in the waters of your womb and the hands, the little fingers and the fingernails. You might even choose to see whether your baby is a girl or a boy. Imagine the umbilical cord floating in the waters of your womb connected to a healthy placenta, supplying the nourishment your baby needs to grow strong and healthy. And as you feel your baby moving, imagine these movements in your mind also. Spend as much time as you wish absorbed in the wonder of this new life with thoughts of love and welcome to your baby.

Colour can be used during this meditation, so visualise a loving colour embracing your baby, a colour that represents the feelings you are wanting to share with your baby.

This meditation also provides the opportunity to acknowledge the transformations that are taking place moment to moment for you, as well as your baby as you both prepare for life after birth. It can be practised as a full meditation on its own or more informally when you simply turn your attention inwards for some special time with your baby. Be as creative as you want to be,

these are unique moments and some of life's most precious. They enable you to appreciate this transient time, and to be ever mindful of the joy of being a woman and now a mother.

As you relax into the meditation know your baby can feel your thoughts, hear the sound of your heartbeat and your breathing, and feel the waters of your womb moving as you breathe, ever so gently. You might like to hum as you do this visualisation, aware that the sound and its healing vibrations gently massage and caress your baby.

And after the birth, among all the busyness of life, remember to make the time to simply be with each other as often as possible. Maybe give your baby a gentle massage after the bath or have a warm bubble bath together. Or indulge yourself by doing nothing other than just watching your beautiful baby sleep. You will soon discover how quickly the days pass and your baby changes, almost before your eyes.

Bec, one of my students, told me how she used the image of her baby in her womb to help during labour. Focusing on the ultrasound of her baby at 20 weeks helped her stay in touch with what was happening beyond the intensity of her contractions. This is a very real and insightful way to be connected with your baby through the birthing process.

Your Baby's Light: The Camera Lens

Sometimes a woman can be in active labour for many hours only to find that her cervix has dilated no more than 3 or 4 centimetres. If labour continues in this way, medical intervention becomes a real possibility.

When the mind holds the idea of birthing the light of your baby's soul—not instead of, but as well as the physical form—you will feel it in your body too. Many women have told me how including this idea in their meditation really helped to change their focus, from just how *big* the baby is … how *big* the head is … how will it possibly fit … to bringing their awareness to birthing the *little* person their baby really is. And sometimes, in a mysterious way, the cervix responds to their thoughts and the 'light' emerging from inside the womb, and opens to the birth. I am not suggesting that this visualisation will make every woman dilate as she wishes, but it is worth trying in preparing your body for birth—to open to the process through this type of visualisation while you are pregnant. It is well accepted that the mind and our will are a very powerful force, and even though there is no real proof that this idea of 'light' actually works, it definitely alters a woman's perception and can be the catalyst for changing the way labour progresses.

Even though it is logical that your baby is a person inside its body, encouraging women to birth their baby, body and soul, has often had a remarkably positive influence. It is a concept they have been able to incorporate very easily as they progress through labour and is especially powerful when their birth supports encourage them to stay focused on that. They are then in communication with their whole baby, physically and mentally, in union with it—mind to mind, body to body, moving through labour together for the gift of life at the moment of birth. Soul to soul. Just as a flower opens to the light from the sun, the cervix can be visualised as softening to your baby's 'light'. It is this soul light that begins to emerge through the cervix and into the world, in the same way that the lens of a camera gradually dilates and opens to allow light into the camera.

Visualising your baby as light can be done as soon as you know your baby is there within you. In the last weeks of your pregnancy do this daily and imagine the cervix gradually becoming ripe and soft, including a colour as well if that feel right for you, so that when labour begins you are ready, body and mind.

The Flower Meditation

In some European cultures it is common to have beautiful flowers around in the last weeks of pregnancy and especially in the room of the birthing woman, as a way of reminding her to open to the birth of her baby as a flower opens to the sun. This has been a welcome thought to many of

the women I see, who include a real or even an artificial flower among the things to remember for birth. Even if the flower is forgotten they still have the image and what it symbolises in their mind.

You might like to imagine that your womb is like a flower bud, with about 40 layers of petals, the petal tips overlapping at your cervix. Your baby is nurtured inside this beautiful bud which is filled with the light from your baby's soul. As your pregnancy progresses, imagine that with each week a layer of petals dissolves, so that for example at 30 weeks pregnancy you have just 10 layers left. The stem of the flower bud is at the top of the womb and reaches into your heart centre, so that your feelings of love can flow from your heart to your baby. This is a powerful birth preparation to use throughout pregnancy.

In the last weeks of your pregnancy as the layers of petals lessen, you might like to imagine the light from your baby creating a soft glow through the petals—like holding a torch on the palm of your hand.

When you are at full term and the birth is imminent you can imagine the last layer of petals, the tips just meeting at the cervix, so you are mentally prepared for labour through visualisation. Feel a warm glow there from your baby as the cervix begins to soften and ripen for birth.

The flower can be brought to mind as you begin labour; it can act as a potent symbol as you move through the birthing process. A flower represents being open

to birthing your baby, just as it opens to the sun. If you enjoy this meditation and relate to what is symbolises, remember to tell your birth support so that they can encourage you to draw on it.

The First Embrace

During pregnancy, despite planning ahead, preparing the nursery, buying clothes and so on, it is sometimes hard to comprehend that at the end of this time you will have your baby in your arms at the beginning of remarkable journey. There are so many changes and so much information to cope with that to actually imagine seeing your baby for the first time can be lost. In the last weeks of your pregnancy it is very important to visualise those first glorious moments together using this creative and intimate meditation.

Concentrate on the actual place where you are planning to birth your baby because this will create a more realistic atmosphere in the meditation. Become relaxed and still, following the flow of your natural breath quietly moving in and out of your body. Clear the environment of your mind of all other thoughts and when

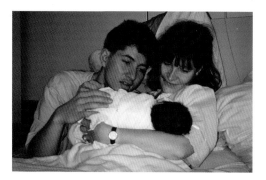

you are ready, imagine you are in the place you have chosen for the birth.

With you are all those people you have asked to be there for the birth of your baby, to nourish and care for you and to love you—your partner, birth supports, doctor and midwife, perhaps your mother or sister. Feel safe, secure and completely supported by these people. Imagine the atmosphere of the room is calm, quiet and peaceful and filled with love for you and your baby. Feel very comfortable and relaxed as you visualise this place. You might like to imagine a beautiful colour filling the room, surrounding all who are there, bringing feelings of love, joy and welcome.

Now visualise your newborn baby resting in your arms for the first time and feel her weight in your arms. See your baby's face and features, observe the tiny movements, look at the beautiful little fingers, hear the new sounds of your baby breathing. Touch your baby's skin and feel how soft and smooth it is. As you absorb all these images and feelings look into your baby's eyes and simply fall in love with each other. Hold these mental pictures in your mind acknowledging the absolute wonder of the moment, so precious, so tender. In your visualisation you might like to include your partner and others who are special to you and your baby, there to love and welcome your baby into the world. A beautiful colour or light can also be seen to surround all of you, illuminating the image and enhancing the feelings you most want to create.

It is worthwhile making a drawing of this image, as I suggest in 'Art therapy' (in chapter 17). This is a beautiful creative way of bringing these precious thoughts into life, which you can keep as a memento of this amazing time in your life. Years after the birth, women often tell me they still have their meditation drawings from pregnancy and that they a very precious memory. This visualisation is best done in the last weeks of your pregnancy.

The Moon and the Water

Throughout history the moon has been associated with women, and comparisons made between the menstrual cycle and the phases of the moon. Menstrual bleeding was often referred to as the 'lunar blood'.

In ancient times women's cycles were balanced and in harmony with the world they lived in and were influential in the creation of the first calendars. *Menses* is the Latin word for 'menstruation' and also means 'month'. As the 28-day phases of the moon offered insight into establishing a system of months and years, so too the female cycle provided a precise way of marking the passing of time. This led to a greater understanding of nature's rhythms, and of women themselves. People all over the world have lived by the phases of the moon using it as a guide to choose the best time to plant or harvest, and even when to fish for the most abundant and best-tasting catch.

The Moon-goddess created time, with its cycles of creation, growth, decline and destruction, which is why ancient calendars were based on phases of the moon and menstrual cycles.
Barbara Walker, *The Women's Encyclopedia of Myths and Secrets*, page 670

Many ancient civilisations have myths describing the mystery of creation, its association with the moon and of the blood women either shed in cycles or were able to 'miraculously' retain for approximately ten moons and thus bring to form a new life. They believed that the cessation of menstrual bleeding and the retention of blood resulted in a baby taking form in the womb.

Just as the moon appears to us to move from being dark and vacant at the new moon, to being completely whole and light at the full moon, so too a woman might intuitively feel a symbolic space and void, an emptiness within herself at the completion of her bleeding, and just prior to her menstruation experience a wholeness and fullness like the fullest moon, as her body prepares to shed the menstrual blood. At the end of her pregnancy a woman is full and luminous like a full moon, carrying within her the light of her unborn baby. After the birth she is again empty.

Some women believe that if a woman conceives in a particular phase of the moon her labour will commence at the same moon time, and this has proven correct for many women.

Water, the other potent symbol in this meditation, is also considered feminine in principle. Water has always been a symbol of great spiritual relevance and referred to as the giver of life. Just as the first life forms on our planet evolved in the vast oceans, so too the baby develops and matures in the waters of a woman's womb, and is therefore significant to this meditation.

All women, but especially pregnant women, enjoy the Moon and Water meditation. The combination of the two symbols makes them feel complete as they take qualities from both to find the symmetry between what is above and what is below—balancing heaven and earth.

Women move into this meditation with a unique knowing and it really seems to be quite specific for them. As the birth draws closer it illustrates in a lovely symbolic way their fullness of body with child and the soft luminosity they all have, like the moon.

Sometimes a woman might not be able to fully embrace her beauty at this time, but when she aligns herself with the qualities of the moon and the water and perceives she has this same radiance within her through the meditation, it encourages her to love and honour herself more easily. Often it can shift the awareness away from what is displeasing to her to embracing the beauty and characteristic glow of a woman carrying a child.

So imagine that you are standing in a beautiful place at the water's edge, in the full moonlight. This source of water might be a lake, the ocean, a cool deep pool in the forest or maybe you are beside a river …

You are standing naked enjoying the soft breeze on your body, and you see the delicate glow of the moonlight on you, caressing the beautiful curves of your pregnant body …

You feel very much a woman in 'full bloom' and you smile to yourself, acknowledging this is a precious and transient moment, loving how you feel and look at this brief moment in your life …

Continue to imagine yourself there in the moonlight breathing in deeply and drawing in the atmosphere of this lovely place …

You see the water before you, calm, clear and still—you can smell and taste the air. You become completely absorbed in the wonder of this beautiful place in nature …

You see the luminous glow of the moonlight on the water leading right up to where you are standing, and you step into the water along the moonbeam, feeling it around your ankles, the water is the perfect temperature and you enjoy the softness of the earth beneath your feet …

You become submerged in the crystal clear water, and instinctively allow yourself to float, light and relaxed in the water …

You are safe in this 'moon water' and feel completely supported by it, feeling the water all around your body and the moonlight glowing translucent on your full belly and your breasts. Look up into the night sky and into the face of the luminous full moon and into the vast, unlimited sky above you, the ageless, infinite space of the universe …

The glow of the moon is on your body and all around you giving the water a light and luminous quality. You feel wonderful as you float and relax deeply in the water. Bring to mind the feminine principles of water and the relevance of the moon to you as a pregnant woman and to your baby in your womb, and truly embrace the beauty of your body …

You might notice there are flowers in the water floating there with you, or sea birds, dolphins and even whales—hear them singing to you and your baby as they sing to their own young—you are in union with these great gifts of nature …

As you gaze into the night sky see it filled with stars and planets giving brightness to the black velvet sky, reaching your awareness far out into that eternal, timeless space. This moment exist only for you, as you float gently in the water, just as your baby is floating in the waters of your womb … and imagine your baby can also feel the same soft moonlight through your body reaching them in your womb.

As you quietly rest in your meditation continue to breathe gently allowing yourself to relax deeper and deeper with each breath, feeling any left over tensions in the physical body gradually dissolving and being replaced with softness, while any unwanted thoughts and feelings disappear from the mind so it becomes clear and calm. Feel cleansed and purified by the meditation.

This image can be held for as long as you like. When you are ready imagine yourself drifting to the water's edge once more, slowly coming out of the water to sit quietly on the shore, allowing your body to dry in the moonlight, or there might be a beautiful gown or robe waiting there for you, like a symbolic gift from the meditation. Rest there for a moment and continue to look out at the moon's reflection on the water. Women are never really ready to come away from this meditation because they embrace it so well, and it is ideal to do on a full moon.

The Chakra Meditation

As a woman progresses through the months of her pregnancy she seems to move inwards to a quieter, less social place within herself and almost without conscious intention she becomes more internalised, focusing more on herself and the baby in her womb and becoming more intuitive. Pregnant women are drawn to this meditation, which I have designed around the traditional chakra meditation. It has grown into a beautiful meditation

and enables women to connect with their innermost, spiritual self and quite simply describes how each chakra has relevance for them and their baby in utero.

To discuss the chakras fully is an in-depth study. Many books have been written about their relevance to the spiritual self and the effects they have on the health and function of the physical body. The brief details here are sufficient for the purpose, but you might like to seek more information.

The word *chakra* means 'wheel' or 'vortex'. Chakras are invisible wheels of spiritual energy located along the inner side of the spinal column on *sushumna nadi*, the main psychic channel in the spiritual body. There are seven major charkas, located in succession from the base of the spine, the seventh chakra is at the top of the head .When they are used in meditation and yoga practices the flow of energy or prana is stimulated. Generally the colours of the rainbow are used for the chakras but I prefer the traditional tantric colours, which differ slightly. Most people seem to relate very well to these colours, even more so than to the rainbow colours. However, keep in mind that if you 'see' colours other than those I suggest this is fine—it is a meditation practice and a very intuitive one, so you should go with what feels right for you in that moment.

Before you begin, relax and settle your mind with some yoga breathing exercises. When you are ready bring your awareness to the base of the spinal

column where *mooladhara*, the base or root chakra, is located. This chakra is associated with the physical energy and vitality, and governs the lower part of the body including the cervix and pelvic floor. When the base chakra is balanced we feel strong, grounded and courageous within ourselves. The colour is brilliant red, the deep blood red of life's energy, the colour of strength, vitality, anger and emotion, power and robust health. This chakra's specific association with pregnancy is the cervix. This is the primal energy centre in a woman's body and what is grounding for birth. Meditating on this, visualising the richness of the colour and its associated strength will enable you to call on this knowledge to assist you mentally and physically in the birthing process. Breathe naturally with your whole awareness at the base chakra. It is also where *kundalini shakti*, our primal energy, is located; one of the aims of yoga is to activate this energy.

Now bring your attention to the second chakra, *swadhisthana*, at the top of the pubic bone, just above the base chakra. The colour is orange. It is associated with pleasure and joy, and the reproductive system, and has an influence on sexual energy and general wellbeing. It is particularly relevant to pregnant women, being the area where the ovaries and the uterus are located. The colour can be seen as a merging of the red of the base chakra and the yellow of the third chakra at the abdomen. *Swadhisthana* is at the point where the qualities from these three centres are concentrated and come together in pregnancy and childbirth. Because the three lower chakras are about the reproductive system and the womb, women are naturally drawn to them in pregnancy and often use these aspects of the meditation during the birthing process. Hold your awareness there, visualising the colour orange while breathing quietly.

Now move your attention to the level of the navel where the third chakra is located. This chakra is called *manipura* and the colour is yellow. *Manipura* is the centre of our personal power and emotional energy it is here that we feel strong emotions. Yellow is associated with joy and life. Imagine it inside your womb, feel the warmth and glow like beautiful sunshine, visualising lovely golden rays all around your baby. Breathe gently and feel the expansion and contraction of your abdomen and be aware of your baby bathing in this lovely glow.

The fourth chakra is *anahata*, at the heart centre. The colour is a beautiful blue that expresses the unconditional feelings of compassion and love you have for yourself and for your baby. Blue is associated with purity, peace, calmness, truth and devotion and is the colour of the mother, the one who nurtures, and in the Christian tradition with Mary, the mother of Jesus. Concentrating at the heart centre is a nourishing and gentle way to honour yourself as a mother. It reminds you that you are precious in your feminine beauty,

you are the one who bears and brings forth new life into the world. *Anahata* is the central place in your spiritual body— feel energy flowing from it to your mind and down into your womb. Breathe gently and feel each breath carrying with it a warmth of love for yourself and for your baby. As you contemplate the heart chakra feel you are receiving blessings from the symbolic mother or from Mary.

From the heart centre move your attention to the throat, to *vishuddhi*, where the colour is purple. This part of your body is associated with communication and self-expression, with speech and voice. Through conscious mediation on the throat centre these aspects will become more balanced and will assist you to harmonise the way you communicate with others. Purple is often considered to be a principal spiritual colour and to be the highest mystical colour. When purple is used specifically for meditation it significantly enhances the quality of the meditations. It is often the colour people 'see' when they first begin visualisation and meditation practices. The throat chakra is at a point in the body that is above the chakras that are more physical in nature, yet it is still below the eyebrow centre, the centre of the conscious/ unconscious mind, the doorway to the infinite mind. When we view the throat chakra in this way it is like the gateway between the physical and earthly, and the mind and the higher consciousness. *Vishuddhi* reminds women to work with

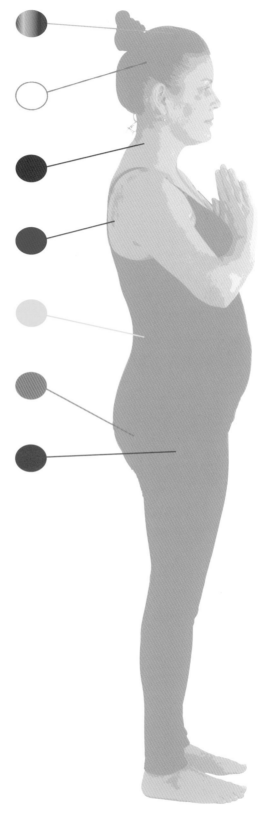

their conscious mind and the physical body, together and in union. Ujjayi breathing is felt at this chakra and for all these reasons is invaluable during childbirth. Ujjayi and humming are specific practices for balancing this chakra and are beneficial for problems associated with the neck, the throat, the thyroid and parathyroid glands.

The next charka, *ajna*, is at the eyebrow centre. This important chakra is known as the 'eye of knowledge and intuition' and rests at the doorway between the conscious and the unconscious mind. It is often referred to as the third eye being linked with psychic ability and clairvoyance and is associated with the qualities of intuition, inner knowing, wisdom and states of higher awareness. This chakra is seen as a sliver, luminous sphere, like a full moon, glowing softly at the centre of the forehead. Rest your awareness there and experience the quiet and peace of the conscious mind just beyond your thoughts. When you hold your awareness there, even if only for a moment, you glimpse the true nature of your mind, which is always clear and luminous. Because your awareness is at the mind centre and the symbol is the moon, meditation on this chakra enables pregnant women to align with their feminine wisdom.

The seventh chakra rests above the top of the head. It is the crown chakra, *sahasrara*. It attributes are beyond the physical body and some say it

is like resting your awareness in the heavenly realms. Swami Satyananda says 'it is the highest psychic centre, the threshold between psychic and spiritual realms which contains all the chakras below it' (*Kundalini Tantra*, page 332). Sometimes it is visualised as purple but from a traditional sense it is seen as multicoloured, carrying all the colours of the spectrum and all their healing vibrations. It is the way to the higher realms, the higher consciousness, to 'god' or the divine energy.

Hold your awareness on these colours and the parts of your body they correspond to, and be aware also of the one or more most prominent for you.

There is a connection between the base chakra and the eyebrow centre chakra that is relevant as a birth preparation, in a purely spiritual sense. Kriya Yoga is a traditional practice based on the chakras in which, when working on the eyebrow centre chakra, practices that relate to the base chakra are included. From a yogic perspective the pelvic floor exercises include *ashwini mudra* or tightening of the anus, and *moola bandha*, the contraction of the perineum, vagina and cervix. *Moola bandha* is a specific practice to balance the eyebrow centre chakra. Simply put, every time you do the pelvic floor exercises you are also working from a spiritual perspective, on the eyebrow centre. Your focus on the cervix and perineum has obvious relevance to birth, while preparing your mind is equally important.

You want to be clear, calm and present in your mind during childbirth. The mind-body connection is what conscious birthing is about and what will benefit you the most in labour. In a purely spiritual and yogic sense, the pelvic floor exercises are a positive way of bringing greater clarity and awareness to your mind, which might encourage their more diligent practice.

All colours have their own unique healing qualities and they can be used in many different situations to assist with healing, to emphasise a particular feeling or to establish balance in the body and mind. They can enhance moods and affect the atmosphere of the mind and emotions in a positive way, often bringing about healing and change.

During labour you can visualise a colour or light in the birth canal as you imagine your baby moving easily and gently to be born. Imagine a beautiful colour around the cervix, at the base charka, as you visualise it gradually opening for the birth of your baby. When your baby is born, visualise a beautiful colour completely surrounding you, your new baby and your birth support. This image applies to every birth, whatever the circumstances.

Spinal Column Meditations

Using awareness of the spinal column as a form of meditation is one of the best practices for improving concentration. This can be approached in a number of different ways, from simple breath awareness up and down your spine, to more elaborate visualisations incorporating colour. I discuss the basic practice, and a few variations that have proven both inspiring and effective for my students.

Before you begin the meditation spend about 10 minutes quietening your mind and becoming still, perhaps using the Breath Balancing posture with either the natural breath, ujjayi or humming.

When you are ready, direct your awareness to the spinal column and as you breathe in, move your awareness from the base of your spine to the top of your head. As you breathe out, move your awareness down again to your tail bone.

Continue with this practice, feeling the breath and prana moving up and down your spine. You will become very conscious of your inner self and notice a feeling of steadiness and strength in your physical posture. This exercise establishes a very firm concentration in the mind and one-pointed awareness.

A visualisation can be included by imagining light or colour within your spinal column, moving up and down with your breath. You might also like to imagine that the colour and your awareness in taken down into the earth, to ground and anchor you in your physical body. This provides a feeling of strength in your physical self and a firm confidence that is valuable if you are very restless, or in adrenal overload and exhausted.

The colour can then be carried through the body and out beyond the top of your head, as if to take your awareness beyond your thoughts and into a peaceful space, to the realm of the higher consciousness. This visualisation is both centring and stabilising—giving a real steadiness in the physical sense, combined with a clear, luminous and present mind state. If you want to proceed more slowly or find it confusing to combine the visualisation with your breathing, let go of breath awareness and just imagine the colour moving through your body more slowly.

The Earth: Your Favourite Place in Nature

Our Earth is often referred to as Mother Earth, the symbolic mother, the one who nurtures, protects and provides nourishment to all living things. It has always been associated with creation, fertility and nourishment, the giver of life—and so the association with women who are also nurturers and give life through pregnancy.

During the last weeks of pregnancy it is quite natural to find yourself becoming more forgetful or vague, less interested in the outside world, withdrawing more into yourself and to your baby in the womb. Although this vagueness is not always a welcome feeling it is quite common, being nature's way of helping you to retreat inward in preparation for birth and becoming a mother. The Earth Meditation is ideal for this time as it has a stabilising

and grounding influence and symbolically helps to bring you in touch with your physical self, with your body and your baby. It is nourishing and replenishing and gives the feeling of being strong and connected to the physical so important during the birthing process.

Simply imagine that you are in one of Earth's special places, one that makes you feel peaceful and connected to your feminine energy. This might be the same beautiful place in nature you would use for one of the other meditations, or it might be somewhere quite different. See this place very clearly in your mind, beginning with the time of day or night. Is this place influenced by the seasons? Open your senses to what you would see and the sounds you would hear, the taste and smell of the air. Feel the earth beneath your body and as you breathe in feel you are drawing the energies from deep in the earth into your whole body, feel yourself becoming steady, strong and connected to the earth and what it represents symbolically.

Now take your awareness to the sky above you. Imagine you are drawing clarity, knowledge and wisdom into mind from the unlimited expanse of the sky. Lift your awareness up to the sun and draw on its radiance and golden colour. The earth can be seen as a symbolic reflection of our physical self, while the sky represents the mind as well as the divine and spiritual aspects of our natures, bringing balance to the physical and spiritual through this visualisation. Relax deeply into this peaceful meditation as a practice on its own, or use it as a basis for another one, such as the Tree or the Mountain.

You might like to imagine a beautiful waterfall in this place, that you stand under it to feel cleansed by the healing water. This can be carried through to when you are having a shower at home or even during labour where time

under a shower is soothing. The shower symbolically washes away all doubt and fear and can be seen as cleansing to your mind, your body and your spirit.

Some women also like to include the image of a cave in their nature setting. A cave can create a very intimate atmosphere, a private inner sanctuary, a safe place to retreat to. Your meditation cave is a place to feel quiet and at peace

with yourself, to contemplate and reflect—for some it has the ambience of the womb, where you can feel safe and nourished just as your baby does in your womb.

The Fire Meditation: Releasing and Cleansing

I have been encouraged to include this meditation by a number of women who have found it very helpful during their pregnancies and at other times. More a creative visualisation than a true meditation, it takes you on an inner journey, in this case one of releasing and cleansing. It follows on from the Earth meditation and can easily be incorporated into it. Its basic principle is to hold onto only what nourishes us and throw out or burn what is limiting in some way. The purpose of this creative exercise is to free ourselves of outmoded thinking and negative beliefs through the cleansing and purifying element of fire.

Imagine you are in your place in nature in the middle of the night, with a clear sky and a full moon so the atmosphere is quiet, still and private. Reflect on any limiting beliefs that are worrying you and possibly holding you back in some way—fears, doubts, insecurities. Make a circle of stones on the ground and gather twigs and sticks to build a safe fire. Light the fire, relax for a while as you watch it burn. You have with you some paper and a pen and you begin to put down what you want to be free of, mentally and emotionally. There might be only one

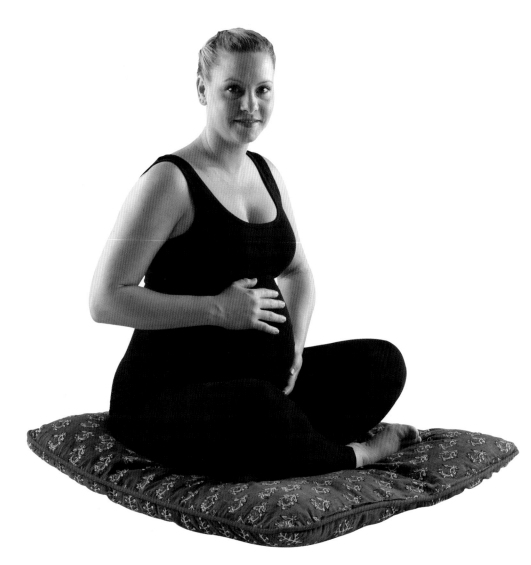

thing or many that you want to release; these may be seen as words or in symbolic form. When you are ready place the paper in the fire and watch it burn—fire is a cleansing and purifying symbol and here you are watching it completely consume your unwanted thoughts and feelings. Take as long as you need, watch the fire dim and finally go out. By now it is dawn in your visualisation, signalling the coming of a new day. Gather the ash from the circle of stones and carry it to a high place, at the edge of a canyon or a cliff, and as the sun comes up open your hands and allow a cool breeze to blow away the last particles of ash, symbolically releasing your unwanted beliefs. Nearby is a cool stream—wash your hands and enjoy this new day and new way of thinking, feel a lightness within yourself and a new freedom.

The various symbols and images in this visualisation are simple, yet very purifying and can be done in relation to birth and becoming a new mother or for any other situation in your life. The results are sometimes very profound and healing to the spirit. After the meditation, write these thoughts down and burn them safely to fully appreciate the value of this meditation. I often suggest this be a ritual at the beginning of a new year, on your birthday or maybe at spring time.

The Tree Meditation

A tree is 'the embodiment of life, the point of union of the three realms, heaven, earth and water' (David Fontana, *The Secret Language of Symbols*, page 100).

I first came across the Tree Meditation in Phyllis Krystal's *Cutting the Ties that Bind*; she used it to encourage confidence and improve self-esteem in her clients. Trees are incredibly beautiful. They give us constant beauty and are a special treasure, providing food, shelter and medicines to humanity and the other creatures of the earth. Most significantly, without trees our planet and all living things would die.

The tree is a symbol of life in many cultures. The Buddha became enlightened while sitting under a bodhi tree in India. In ancient times trees were objects of worship to the druids and other peoples. In some Middle Eastern countries there were 'sacred groves in which to practise phyllomancy, the art of divination by listening to the rustling of leaves' (Barbara Walker, *The Women's Dictionary of Symbols and Sacred Objects*, page 202). This is a lovely thought for a meditation and can easily be done if you are able to meditate in a natural setting and focus on the wind moving in the trees.

The evergreen tree represents a healthy life, abundance and prosperity; the deciduous tree, in reflecting the cycle of the seasons, represents birth, life, death and rebirth. In summer, the deciduous tree is full with abundant growth; in autumn the leaves change and die as the days become cooler and there is less light. Winter is a time for inner growth, regeneration and preparation for rebirth

of the tree's energy, followed by signs of new life in the spring. The tree is a potent symbol of strength, stability, nurturing and grace.

The Tree Meditation provides a feeling of inner strength and quiet confidence to help women cope with the many changes, fears and doubts that can surface as pregnancy progresses. It is particularly recommended for those who feel unsure of their ability to cope during labour or as a mother, and for those who are not completely happy about the changes in their pregnant bodies and may have lost their usual self-confidence and joy in life. It is also valuable after the birth when everything is new and often overwhelming.

The tree is seen to stand strong between heaven and earth. This meditation can be practised in your usual place for meditation, but you might also like to sit against a tree in a forest or one in your garden.

Spend a little time quietening your mind and becoming still. When you are relaxed and centred, visualise yourself standing before a fully grown, healthy tree—perhaps one that is familiar to you, a tree you have seen in a photo or an imaginary tree with magical qualities. Visualise the tree in all its beauty standing firmly in the ground. See the height of the tree, the trunk, the branches and the leaves. Imagine the earth below the tree, and the sun shining directly above, giving light and warmth to tree and earth.

When you are ready, go to the tree and lean against it with your arms outstretched, feeling how easily it takes your weight and supports you. Then sit on the ground with your spine against the trunk, feeling safe and secure.

Bring your attention to the ground beneath you and visualise the roots of the tree spreading deep and wide and holding the tree firmly. Imagine the roots seeking nutrients deep in the earth. Know that the earth has provided all that the tree has needed, from the time it was a seed to full maturity as you see it in your meditation. As you breathe in, feel you are drawing into yourself the earth's energies. These are the energies of the symbolic mother nourishing you with the love, tenderness and reassurance to help you feel strong and secure within yourself. As you breathe out, release all the doubts and insecurities from within.

Now visualise the sun above the tree and feel the warmth of its rays. Imagine the sunlight shining on the leaves and branches; be aware that the sun has provided the tree with the light and warmth to grow tall and strong. As you breathe in, imagine you are drawing energy from the sun; feel the warmth giving you energy and clarity. Think of all the qualities a father gives a child, such as confidence, courage and wisdom, and draw them in with each breath. As you breathe out, release all uncertainty and fear and other limiting beliefs. Continue for as long as you wish before

simply reflecting on the qualities of the meditation.

The Wish-fulfilling Tree

When I first introduced this meditation, I was surprised at how much the women in my classes enjoyed it and benefited from it. They said it encouraged them to have real goals about their pregnancies and birthings, and about becoming a mother. It gave them the opportunity to explore how they felt, and what they really wanted at this special time in their lives.

The wish-fulfilling tree can be a tree in your garden or in a forest, a tree you are quite familiar with. However, as this particular tree has magical qualities and will carry your dreams and wishes, you might like to imagine something more creative, or not quite of this world. A Christmas tree, including the star at the top, is often used.

In your mind see the tree standing majestic and strong. You can imagine brilliant sunshine giving light and warmth to your tree, or maybe gentle moonlight making your tree glow, luminous and soft. Imagine you are either leaning up against your tree or gazing at it from a distance. Make a wish concerning your pregnancy and visualise it on the tree as a coloured ball or a beautiful coloured light. Use your imagination—your wishes can be seen in whatever way feels the best for you. Continue making wishes about your labour and the birth, and maybe another about your first moments together with

your baby, or being a mother in the early weeks of your baby's life. This is a tree of abundance and the number of wishes you place on it is unlimited.

Sometimes you will make only one or two wishes, other times the whole tree will be filled with your fondest dreams. See the sun or the moon shining a radiance and glow on your wishes as if to give blessings to them. An affirmation might come to mind that encompasses the feelings expressed in your wishes, something you can repeat to yourself daily to remind you of your meditation.

When you have finished just allow the tree to dissolve into the light as a way of letting your wishes go—completely detached from them and trusting they will manifest in your life in the most appropriate way.

This meditation can be done about any aspect of your life, and at any time in your life. I often suggest doing it at the beginning of a new year, or on your birthday, to set in place some of your intentions for the months and years to come. I suggest you draw your tree to remind you of your precious dreams, which you can refer to throughout the year. Many times the wishes start to come true, in the perfect way and at the perfect time.

The Mountain

Sit, then, as if you were a mountain, with all the unshakeable, steadfast majesty of a mountain.

Sogyal Rinpoche, *Meditation*, page 35

When I use the image of a mountain for meditation, most people relate to it very easily, with excellent results. Mountains have always been symbols of great power, indomitable energy and enormous beauty; they can have an almost god-like presence. We are fascinated by their seemingly invincible force, in awe of their extraordinary beauty and incredible atmosphere. Being in the mountains can be a dynamic and emotional experience, both when the elements are at their most volatile and fervent, and when they are still and silent.

Mountains have been chosen as places of retreat by masters of meditation and devout yogis who spend many years in uninterrupted solitude. Countless monasteries, temples, shrines and other religious monuments have been constructed high in mountainous landscapes—the belief being that the higher the mountain, the closer are the heavenly realms and the deities of worship. Mountains have been said to be the meeting places of heaven and earth. The earth-bound base of the mountain relates to our physical reality, the top of the mountain reaching towards heaven represents our spiritual natures and aspirations.

When you are seated in a traditional cross-legged posture, your body in silhouette resembles the shape of a mountain, wide at the base and tapering to a peak at the top of your head. The image of the mountain will make you feel extremely still, steady, solid—in your body and your mind. It provides you with all the feelings symbolised by mountains and is very helpful if you need to feel more grounded and strong. It is also an excellent image to bring to mind to improve self-esteem and create more self-confidence. You might see yourself on the mountain or see yourself as the mountain—both will bring you the empowering feelings represented by the mountain.

See all your unwanted thoughts swirling around your head in the same way that wind, snow and sleet rage around the top of a mountain. Like a steady mountain, you are not disturbed or moved by all this mental activity; no matter how strong the distraction or how severe the storm you remain firm in yourself.

See the wind decreasing as your thoughts subside and the sun shining brilliantly in an azure sky, bringing clarity and illumination to your mind. Or imagine that it is midnight, and as the snow and sleet disappear the sky is like black velvet filled with stars; a brilliant full moon shines luminous over the mountain, bringing enrichment and clarity to your thoughts.

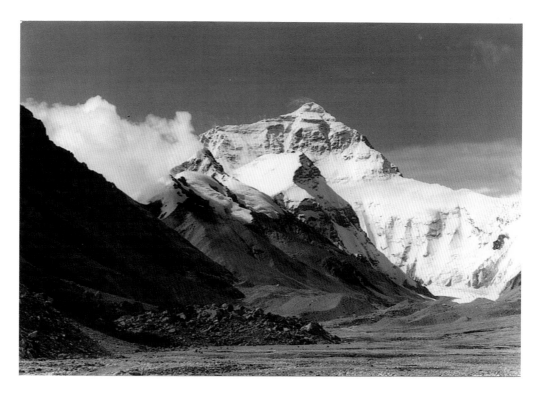

The Golden Spiral

The Golden Spiral is similar to the Mountain meditation in that you are sitting in the shape of an inverted V, where the form is wide at the base and comes to a peak at the top. You will feel grounded and connected to the earth—strong in your physical self and peaceful in your mind. I have watched people during this practice and they actually sit taller and lift their heads higher as the spiral formation is visualised soaring above them.

Always begin your meditation becoming quiet and still. When you are ready, visualise yourself in a beautiful place in nature, a vast open space. Now imagine you are sitting inside a golden circle, which can be as large or small as you like. A circle represents unbroken energy because it has no beginning or end, just continuous energy, and is often considered to be perfect and eternal. The circle is a feminine symbol. It is protective and is associated with equality and balance. In Western culture, many of these meanings come together in the wedding ring, which is traditionally gold and represents unbroken love.

Slowly draw the golden circle upwards so that it begins to form a spiral that gradually moves up and around your body. The spiral will become narrower the higher up your body it moves until it reaches a peak above the centre of your head, like a cone.

Imagine the space inside the spiral is filled with complete balance and harmony.

The energy is of the purest, most peaceful kind. Breathe quietly and gently, enjoy the calmness you feel. You might like to imagine the sun or the moon high above, bringing a radiant and luminous glow all around your spiral and inside it.

This is a wonderful environment in which to repeat your affirmations, and for including other visualisations, especially about your baby in your womb.

When you want to come out of the meditation slowly reverse the spiral formation until you again visualise you are sitting inside a golden circle, or simply allow it to dissolve and find yourself resting once more in your special place in nature.

The Ocean of Abundance

This special visualisation technique comes from Phyllis Krystal's wonderful *Cutting the Ties that Bind*. She calls it 'The Wave for Relaxation'. I have often included it in my classes. Many people have commented on the effectiveness of combining this visualisation with deep breathing for overcoming stress and tension.

The ocean is a symbol of abundance, the salt in the water is a universal cleanser and healer, and the colour is both healing and calming. In this meditation, a slow healing wave of water brings peace, balance and harmony to every aspect of yourself as it washes over you, and takes away with it all physical, emotional and mental stress.

This meditation is ideal when you are having trouble sleeping, or bothered by too many unwanted thoughts or uncomfortable feelings. It is helpful during labour in establishing quietness and calmness between contractions, and especially after the birth if you are exhausted and need to restore your energies. During labour imagine any physical tension, anxiety, fear or restlessness being washed away from you as you breathe out deeply, leaving you revitalised and calm as you prepare for the next contraction.

Begin by lying in a comfortable position, or sitting in your bean bag with your body relaxed and your eyes lightly closed. Imagine you are on a beach, at the water's edge. As you breathe in deeply, imagine a wave moving slowly over your body to the top of your head, bringing with it cleansing, healing and peace.

As you breathe out through your mouth, imagine the wave moving back over your body and out into the ocean, taking with it all physical and emotional tensions, leaving you renewed and refreshed. With each breath feel yourself becoming lighter and more relaxed on every level.

The final two meditations are part of normal daily life put into slow motion, to form very interesting meditations that provide many worthwhile benefits. They incorporate all the principals of meditation and can be instrumental in better understanding the feeling and purpose of meditation. They are always enjoyed and due to their curious nature often result in lively conversation afterwards.

The Sultana Meditation

A couple of years ago I went to a seminar held by inspirational speaker Stewart Wilde where he presented the Sultana Meditation as part of his program to encourage deep concentration and mental clarity. This is an excellent meditation and mindfulness exercise, although definitely not a traditional yoga practice. I am including it because it teaches the concepts of meditation so well. It is an excellent practice for beginners and for those who find it difficult to stay focused.

The sultana (dried grape) becomes your complete point of focus; this helps you to understand what meditation is. Meditation is concentration, contemplation and mindfulness, and in this practice you become completely absorbed by the single sultana. You develop a one-pointed awareness of it and fully experience the present moment. (I am always being asked if it could be done with a chocolate-coated sultana; I haven't tried that yet, but it sounds very appealing.)

This meditation can take 10 minutes, or as long as 20 minutes, and most people find they are able to stay completely absorbed without being distracted. This is quite an achievement as under normal circumstances our attention span is not much more than two minutes. People

are amazed by where the time has gone and how incredible it is to concentrate so deeply on a single sultana for that amount of time. It gives a whole new meaning to eating, the enjoyment of food and the sense of taste.

The purpose of this meditation is to slow right down—the more slowly you proceed the more you will appreciate it and the more internalising it will be. The idea is to lose complete awareness of time and be completely absorbed in the practice.

Sit in a position in which you know you will be able to stay comfortable for at least 15 minutes, with your eyes lightly closed. Place a sultana in the palm of your hand. Become aware of both its lightness and its surprising sense of weight. After some time, place the sultana in your mouth. Very slowly begin to explore its contours, texture, shape and size with your tongue, and feel the movements of your mouth and jaw. Continue doing this for as long as you wish, then place the sultana between your teeth and very, very slowly begin to chew. Experience the explosion of sweetness on your taste buds. Feel your teeth gradually coming together, chewing the sultana as if your world has begun to move in slow motion … like a cow chewing its cud in very slow motion … watch as the sultana begins to change form and texture. You can swallow as you need to throughout the meditation. The sultana will completely transform from

something plump and full, to just a few stringy bits of skin. Finally, swallow the remains of the sultana. Remain focused on the sweet aftertaste until you are ready to come out of the meditation. As an amusing sidelight, some women say after this meditation that they become so attached to their sultana that they really don't want to swallow it! More seriously, this technique has sometimes been used successfully for people suffering from eating disorders.

The Walking Meditation

This Buddhist Walking Meditation practice is very similar in nature to the Sultana Meditation, and the results are quite comparable. In this you simply walk barefoot as slowly as possible, heel–foot–toes, being totally mindful of one foot following the other. You are walking almost at a standstill, only not quite. A distance that would normally take a minute to walk will take 15 minutes, and more. This is an incredibly peaceful meditation practice, a wonderful way to slow right down in your outer and inner worlds. It is tranquillising, mesmerising and amazingly relaxing, like a walking hypnosis. You might do this on a beach, on damp grass or even on a gravel road. Those of you who don't like walking barefoot on a rough surface will be surprised to discover that the ground feels soft and pleasant under your feet, never sharp and painful.

CHAPTER 15
DEEP RELAXATION: YOGA NIDRA

The practice of deep relaxation is integral to all yoga programs and especially valuable during pregnancy and after the birth. It is an excellent way to relax your body, calm your mind and replenish lost energies and in many ways is even more relevant as an antidote to the stresses of modern life than the yoga exercises. The value of spending time in deep relaxation is recognised and recommended by all health care professionals.

When you give yourself some quiet time to relax you are recognising the need to take time out, to nourish yourself and to replenish your energies—and is another way that yoga provides you with some gentle practices that enable you to care for yourself in preparation for childbirth.

What is Deep Relaxation?
Yoga nidra means 'dynamic sleep'. During yoga nidra, the physical body experiences complete relaxation and stillness as if it were sleeping but the mind remains alert and awake. This deep state of mind is much more profound than normal resting states and lies somewhere between being awake and being asleep, somewhere between your conscious and your unconscious mind and far beyond your normal range of awareness. During yoga nidra you move gently into the quieter more peaceful aspects of your self, where the more expansive realms of your mind are revealed.

During deep relaxation your senses are gradually withdrawn from the world around you, you become detached from the outside environment and the usual chatter of your mind. This enables you to rest in a calm, gentle place where true peace and quiet can be found. It is here, in this space deep within your own being, that your most peaceful feelings will be discovered and from where meditation can naturally evolve. This then leads to *samadi*—the fulfilment of meditation. In samadi there is only the experience of joy, pure consciousness and truth, where the practitioner is at one with the object of his or her meditation.

Yoga Nidra is the doorway to Samadi.
Swami Satyananda, *Yoga Nidra, Deep Relaxation*

Samadi is a state of being above mortal existence, of state of union with the object of meditation and universal consciousness.
Swami Satyananda, *Kundalini Tantra,* page 322

[Samadi] is a peace that surpasseth all understanding … the state can only be expressed by profound silence … The Yogi has departed from the material world and is merged in the Eternal.
BKS Iyengar, *Light on Yoga*, page 52

Only by spending time in deep relaxation and then meditation can we begin to glimpse what the great teachers are really describing and encouraging us to realise through these traditional yogic teachings.

The Value of Deep Relaxation
The value of deep relaxation goes beyond relieving fatigue and tiredness. When deep

relaxation is practised regularly, balance is restored in your mind and your body and your energies are replenished. It is nourishing on all levels of your being and enables your mind and body the time to heal more completely, and for good health to be established and maintained. It is a similar concept to power napping, which has been proven to increase alertness, improve concentration and reduce fatigue. As little as 15 minutes of relaxation can remove the mental fogginess that is common mid-afternoon, or the result of over-effort. Time in deep relaxation or in power napping to revitalise themselves is how many people cope with the demands of modern living.

We have become conditioned to pushing ourselves when we are tired, to keep on going even when we are at the point of chronic physical and emotional exhaustion. Often it is not until we are forced to stop, due to the appearance of physical symptoms or signs of emotional stress, that we become more conscious of how we are living our lives. Many people feel guilty if they take time out to relax or to sleep during the day, even when they are totally exhausted. Women, and especially mothers, are particularly prone to succumb to this misplaced notion. If you can establish the habit of spending a short time in relaxation and meditation during pregnancy, there is more chance that you will do it later when you are at home with your baby.

Difficult times occur in every one's life

but through understanding relaxation and some of the other yoga practices you are more likely to stay well and cope better with stress. It is far better to become familiar with relaxation techniques and regularly take time out to re-energise yourself than to wait until exhaustion or illness due to chronic stress take hold. Without deep relaxation, medications often take longer to be effective or merely mask the true cause of the illness. Making relaxation a habit is like having an inbuilt insurance scheme because the more time you invest in maintaining good health on every level and living a more balanced lifestyle, the greater the rewards will be in the long term.

Deep relaxation is especially valuable during pregnancy and after birth as a way to really nourish and care for yourself. Even if you are already very relaxed, someone who rarely gets ruffled or worried, you will still benefit from time in deep relaxation. The value of relaxation becomes even more apparent when your health is compromised—if you are overtired, have high or low blood pressure, suffer from regular headaches or insomnia, or dealing with a stressful situation. It is also an opportunity to spend some quiet moments together with your baby in your womb.

Many of us seek to know peace and calmness and are constantly searching outside ourselves to fulfil those desires and satisfy our restless needs. Through the practice of deep relaxation, and meditation,

we come to realise we need only look outside ourselves for guidance and to learn the recommended skills, as it is within ourselves that true clarity and quietness dwell and where we can become healers to ourselves on every level of our being. Time spent in relaxation and meditation is healing on every level of your being – your mind, your body and your soul.

Relaxation Postures

I have included three relaxation postures that are suitable for pregnancy, all simple to do and very gentle on your body. The position of your body has a big influence on your ability to relax completely, so it is important the select the posture that is most comfortable for you.

The first two postures, the Corpse and the Flapping Fish, can be used during your yoga practices, in bed, or when you need to rest during the day. They are designed to allow your muscles to release tension so that your body begins to feel heavy, sinking into the floor, or light and weightless.

The third posture, the Sleeping Tortoise, is a very effective way to induce a deep mental calmness when you are unsettled and will quieten your mind very quickly. It is recommended here for relaxation but also has great value as a physical exercise. The Sleeping Tortoise gently stretches your spinal column, releases unwanted tension from the lower back and the shoulders, and is very helpful if you have tightness in the neck.

It will be a matter of trying each of these positions to establish which is most comfortable as this will be influenced by the changes in your body and the way your baby is positioned in your womb.

The Child Pose is another excellent position for relaxation and a favourite among pregnant women. I have dedicated a chapter to it because of the many wonderful benefits it provides for the mind and body during pregnancy and childbirth, including modifications so it is suitable for most women.

General Points

- Lie on a soft but firm surface free from draughts and other disturbances.
- Make sure you will be completely comfortable for the intended relaxation time. Use as many cushions as you need.
- If the weather is cool, cover yourself with a blanket as your body temperature will naturally fall when you relax and wear socks as the feet are the first part of the body to feel cool. If possible, remain quite still for the whole relaxation.

- There are many tapes available for the purpose of relaxation. Having one of your own enables you to practise in the comfort and privacy of your home.
- The time given to relaxation can be anywhere from a 10 minutes to half an hour.

The Corpse: *Shavasana*

The Corpse posture is the classic yoga posture for relaxation but during pregnancy it is really only suitable for the first trimester. This is because lying on your back puts pressure on the major vein on the right side of your body, the vena cava, which can often cause nausea and general discomfort. Because of this, always lie with your legs slightly bent, with a cushion under your knees and another under your head. Place a third cushion under your right hip to elevate it slightly and relieve the pressure on the vena cava. This is often enough to overcome any discomfort due to the extra weight on the abdomen. This is important to remember

if you are required to lie on your back for a medical procedure such as an ultrasound which might take 15 minutes or more.

> **Note:** When you come into this position or come out of it always proceed in this way to prevent stain to your abdomen and lower back: from a seated position bend your knees first and then ease yourself to the floor in a sideways movement using your hands for support. To sit up, roll onto your side and use your hands to help you come into a seated position. This technique also applies to sitting up in bed, lying down to sleep, and to the spinal twists practised lying on your back.

1. Lie on a comfortable surface with your head supported on a cushion, your spine straight and your knees slightly bent with a cushion or rolled up towel under them, and another cushion under your right hip. Cover yourself with a light rug. Remember, if you begin to feel uncomfortable always roll off your back and rest on your left side briefly before sitting up.

2. Relax your face and lightly close your eyes. Incline the chin towards the chest to relieve any pressure from your neck. Your teeth are a little apart and your jaw is relaxed. Allow your lips to rest in a soft smile and be sure you are not frowning.

3. Your arms are a little away from your body with your palms turned upwards, your thumbs and index fingers joined in *chin mudra*. If you prefer, place your hands on your abdomen. There is no effort in your body's position and your breathing is quiet and gentle. As you begin to relax, feel peace and calmness moving into your body and your mind.

The Flapping Fish:
Matsya Kridasana

The Flapping Fish is a very comfortable posture to use when the Corpse posture becomes uncomfortable. Many women find that from around 15 weeks pregnancy the Flapping Fish posture is more comfortable for both relaxing and sleeping. It is especially useful if your lower back is sore or if your back muscles are tight.

Rest your head on a cushion, and place another under your bent knee and abdomen to ease pressure on your back. The full body-length pillows available from some department stores and bedding specialists are ideal for this. This posture is particularly beneficial if you have sciatica problems because it relaxes the nerves to your legs. The pelvic area is lightly stretched which gently stimulates your digestive system.

1. Lie on your right side with your head resting on a pillow or along your arm. (You can rest on either side, as your comfort will depend on the position of your baby.)

2. On your right side your right leg is straight and your left leg is bent, your left knee resting on the floor or on a cushion. Your left hand can rest on the floor, or you might like to place your hand on your abdomen to feel your baby in your womb. Adjust your position to give you the most comfort. This is an ideal position for aromatherapy massage either by your birth support or by a massage therapist.

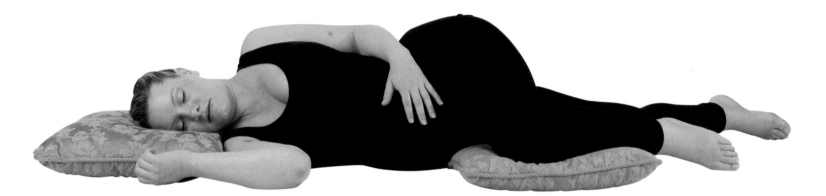

147

The Sleeping Tortoise:
Supta Kurmasana

The Sleeping Tortoise is similar to the Child Pose in that it is very easy to do and is a very suitable relaxation pose for pregnancy. The few women who are not relaxed in the Child Pose will usually find this one to their liking. However, for women who are short in the body or who are carrying their baby high, the Sleeping Tortoise could feel a bit cramped later in pregnancy and should be modified slightly by bending only slightly forward, or placing a semi-filled bean bag between your legs and resting over it. It will be a matter of trying out these positions to establish the most comfortable one to use at different stages.

Many worthwhile benefits are attributed to this easy pose. It will deeply relax your whole body and bring an almost instant calmness to your mind, being a very effective posture for relieving mental and emotional stress. The pelvic area, hips and inner thighs are toned and the abdominal area gently massaged. The longer the posture is held the more your back muscles will soften and relax and your inner thigh area opens so that your body gradually unfolds into the forward bend. The more time spent in this position the closer your head comes towards your feet and the more relaxed you will feel in your body and your mind. As your head is down your mind will quickly relax and even after a short time you might find yourself feeling a little sleepy.

This is a good posture to remember after the birth as well, as it relieves upper back tightness and reduces mental fatigue and other stress.

1. Sit on the floor, on a cushion if you like, with the soles of your feet together, a little further away from your body than in the Butterfly posture. Relax your knees and allow them to fall towards the floor. For more comfort you can place cushions under your knees. Do not force your knees closer to the floor in the Sleeping Tortoise, as this position is more about your body being completely relaxed than flexible.

2. Place your hands on top of your feet, or pass them through your legs to rest beside your feet with your palms facing upwards. Ease your body towards your feet in a gentle forward bend that you can relax deeply into. Relax your head and neck and keep your arms free and loose from your shoulders. The weight of your head will naturally stretch your neck and back so there is no need to ever force your body into the final position. Remember to bend your elbows slightly to prevent tightness in your arms and upper body.

3. Close your eyes and breathe quietly while you hold the posture. Be aware that your back, shoulders, arms and hands are relaxed at all times. As a guide, this can be held for nine breaths but if you're really enjoying it, stay there as long as you remain relaxed and comfortable. Counting your breaths is an excellent way to stay aware of the present while it will improve your concentration skills and therefore prevents your mind from wandering.

CHAPTER 16
SEVEN EASY PROGRAMS

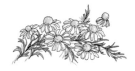

I am often asked for specific, individualised programs that can be done between classes. With so many exercises and practices to choose from, it can become confusing deciding which ones to do, especially if you are new to yoga. A structured, well-balanced program you can follow at home is an ideal way to become familiar with the various techniques, and ultimately to achieve more enjoyment from yoga. The six half-hour programs consist of the gentle exercises, breathing exercises, relaxation and meditation already discussed. Even if you are attending regular classes, it will help to practise yoga at home. These programs are well-balanced, easy to follow mini routines designed for use whenever you have the time or feel inclined to practise yoga.

Once you have the basic format in mind, and recognise how to put it all together, you can then create other programs to suit your own requirements. Follow all the guidelines and precautions and if necessary, adjust what I have proposed to suit your needs. Always remember to be adaptable and flexible with yourself. Sometimes you might feel fatigued and prefer to spend more time meditating or in deep relaxation rather than concentrating on the postures, which is fine.

Backache and other back problems are quite common during pregnancy, so program 7 is included specifically to help alleviate them. For the best results I suggest you practise these postures and exercises as often as possible between your regular classes. They are particularly beneficial when done in conjunction with massage or other treatments for back discomfort.

Getting Started

Always begin with a short relaxation followed by some slow, deep yoga breathing. If you are in the first trimester, lie on your back with your knees bent; further along in your pregnancy lie on your side. Follow the rhythm of your natural breath flowing evenly and gently in and out of your body. Spend between five and ten minutes relaxing and breathing, and getting in touch with your pregnancy and with your baby.

When you are ready, breathe slowly and deeply three or four times. Notice how you are feeling and use your breathing to release any tension or uneasy emotions, replacing them with a more positive atmosphere. Think about how you would prefer to be feeling, and draw in these calming, balancing energies with the breath. When you do this, you will be better prepared for your yoga practice, with a clearer mind and a more centred attitude.

When you are relaxed and centred, proceed with the programs. I suggest also including the pelvic floor exercises (page 84-87) daily, remembering they can be done anywhere and at any time.

Feel free to change the format of these programs and create your own from the many exercises and postures in the book. Most importantly, enjoy your yoga and meditation and the many wonderful benefits it provides.

Program 1

1. Standing and warming up:
   Hand and finger exercises (page 65)
   Shoulder rotations (page 67)
   Head and neck exercises (page 66)
   Pelvic Rocking from a standing position (page 70)
2. The Easy Spinal Twist, waist rotation pose (page 58)
3. The Tree balance and the Dynamic Tree (page 80)
4. The Heavenly Stretch Pose (page 69)
   The Triangle Side Bend (page 71)
   The Warrior (page 75)
   The Hero (page 73)
5. Relaxing: The Child Pose (page 63)
6. Pranayama:
   Deep Cleansing Breaths (page 108)
   Alternate Nostril Breathing (page 101)
   Cooling Breath, including the Breath Balancing Pose if you prefer (page 102)
7. Relaxing:
   Deep relaxation by yourself (page 144), or play a 20-minute relaxation tape

Program 2

1. Standing and warming up:
   Head and neck exercises (page 66)
   Shoulder rotations (page 67)
   Hamstring stretches (page 76)
2. Chest Expansion with deep breathing (page 67)
3. Squatting:
   On a stool and stretching (page 47)
   Squatting from side to side (page 49)
   The moving squat (page 48)
   The Deep Standing Squat (page 51)
   Any other squatting exercises and asanas of your choice.
4. On hands and knees:
   The Cat (page 40)
   Pelvic Rocking (page 37)
   The Tiger (page 42)
5. Relaxation: The Child Pose with variations, including resting over a bean bag (page 63)
6. Pranayama:
   Alternate Nostril Breathing (page 101)
   Ujjayi pranayama (page 106)
   Humming (page 103)
7. Mediation of your choice or deep relaxation.

Program 3

1. Sitting and warming up:
   Exercises for the feet and ankles (page 25)
   Hip rotations (page 27)
   The Half Butterfly (page 28)
   The Butterfly (page 28)
   The Equestrian pose (page 30)

The Sleeping Tortoise, resting on a bean bag if you like (page 148)
2. Seated Spinal Twists: any of the seated or lying down spinal twists (pages 58-62)
3. Pelvic Tilt, then knees to the chest and rocking from side to side (page 43)
4. Pranayama: Any breathing exercises of your choice (pages 95-106)
4. The Candle or other meditation, followed by deep relaxation

Program 4

1. Warming up: Any of the standing warming-up exercises (pages 65-68)
2. Balancing:
   The Tree (page 80)
   The Eagle (page 82)
3. Standing:
   The Wide-A Leg Stretch and variations (page 76)
   The Mountain and variations (page 78)
4. Pelvic rocking (page 70)
5. Relaxation: Child Pose (page 63)
7. Meditation with ujjayi pranayama, and relaxation

Program 5

1. Warming up with any floor exercises of your choice to complement the seated wide leg stretches (pages 31-36)
2. Hip rotations (page 27)
   Half Butterfly (page 28)
   Butterfly (page 28)
3. Seated wide leg posture and variations (pages 31-36)

4. Spinal Twists: any seated or lying down spinal twist of your choice (pages 58-62)

   The Pelvic Tilt, then knees into the chest and rocking from side to side (page 43)

5. Pranayama:

   The Humming Breath (page 103)

   The Cooling Breath (page 102)

   Ujjayi pranayama (page 106)

6. Deep relaxation and the Candle Meditation

Program 6

1. Warming up with floor exercises for the squatting exercises (pages 25-29)

   Squatting postures of your choice (pages 47-53)

   Wall Stretches (the Butterfly, the Squat, the Wide Leg Stretch) (pages 54-55)

2. Spinal Twists: any seated or lying down spinal twists of your choice (pages 58-62)

3. The Cat (page 40)

   The Tiger (page 42)

   Pelvic Rocking (on your knees) (page 37)

4. Relaxation: Child Pose (page 63)

5. Pranayama: three breathing exercises of your choice (pages 95-106)

6. Deep relaxation or meditation

Program 7
Relieving Back Discomfort

This program will only take 10 or 15 minutes and can be followed with relaxation or meditation. If you have back pain do this as often as possible. I have given similar programs to many women and usually the results were noticeable within a very short time. This short program provides the opportunity to relieve discomfort between classes, preventing a constantly aching back and reducing the need for massage or other therapies.

> **Caution:** Always warm up first as directed above, doing a selection from the standing and floor exercises, and take note of any precautions and modifications.

1. Commence on the hands and knees and practice slow Pelvic Rocking, before resting in the Child Pose. Repeat this three times. Follow this with the Cat and the Tiger, followed by more Pelvic Rocking between the exercises.

2. Practise all the seated spinal twists, moving from the easiest to the more advanced postures.

3. Squatting exercises and postures. These are especially valuable as they open into the hips, lower back and pelvic area so well. I suggest commencing with those on a stool first and then progressing through to the others, always noticing how you are feeling and following the precautions and modifications. Even if you are unable to do any more than squat on a stool you will still receive excellent benefits from this position.

   Come onto the hands and knees and practise more Pelvic Rocking and rest into the Child Pose. The Sleeping Tortoise can also be practised as it relieves back and neck discomfort, resting over a bean bag if that gives the most comfort.

4. The standing wide leg stretches give similar benefits. Again, use the stool or rest on something first before continuing onto the full stretch. As with the squatting, the modified variations will greatly relieve your back of discomfort and strain. Leaning against the wall and stretching from that position is wonderful for your legs and back, while the Mountain can be done for a deeper stretch in these parts of your body.

5. From a standing position practise the Easy Spinal Twist and Pelvic Rocking.

6. If you are comfortable resting on your back the Pelvic Tilt is an excellent position to practise regularly. Also include either of the spinal twists from the back, providing they are not causing any discomfort. Rocking on your back with your knees into your chest is a good way to complete the postures on your back. However, be mindful—if your back 'catches' as you rock from side to side, stop rocking. On completion, roll onto your side and come onto the hands and knees. Practice slow Pelvic Rocking and then rest in the Child Pose.

CHAPTER 17

FROM AROMATHERAPY TO CRYSTALS

In this chapter I include a few things which are not yoga but which complement it well to support you in an easier and more relaxed labour and birth.

Aromatherapy Massage

Aromatherapy massage using the essential oils specific to pregnancy is meant to be gentle and nourishing. It has many applications and therapeutic benefits, and a wide range of physical and emotional problems can be relieved when the relevant oils are used, either as a therapy on their own or in conjunction with other remedies. Consult a qualified aromatherapist who will mix the relevant oils for you.

Aromatherapy massage is one of the most wonderful ways to nurture yourself at any time, but especially during pregnancy and as you move through the birthing process. It can be given by a specialist in this field but it is included here as a gentle way for your partner and birth support to pamper you. The technique is simple and easy, and no previous knowledge is needed—the only requirement is a willingness to lovingly support you and offer relief from any discomfort or fatigue you may be feeling.

When you pack your bag for the hospital, remember to take your essential oils with you to help maintain balance and calmness during labour, and to assist relaxation after the delivery.

> **Caution: AVOID** the following essential oils during pregnancy: basil, camphor, cedarwood, chamomile, cinnamon bark, clary sage, clove, fennel, hyssop, jasmine, juniper, marjoram, melissa, myrrh, pennyroyal, peppermint, oreganum, rosemary, sage, thyme and wintergreen.

Essential Oils for Pregnancy

- **Lavender**'s gentle relaxing properties make it a specific for labour and for pain relief.
- **Bergamot** is uplifting and refreshing and reduces stress.
- **Mandarin** and **orange** are uplifting to the mind and spirit, and are effective when added to a carrier oil, such as cold pressed almond oil, for the prevention of stretch marks.
- **Neroli** is also recommended for the skin and is calming and excellent for all stressful situations as well as during recovery.
- **Rosewood** brings clarity to the mind and is useful for the management of stress.
- **Sandalwood** is a beautiful oil which has a very earthy aroma and gives

feelings of courage and emotional strength.

- **Geranium** helps relieve mild anxiety and depression and is uplifting.
- **Ylang-ylang** is calming and relaxing and is recommended for labour.

Essential Oils for Birth

- **Jasmine** is a uterine tonic and is therefore *not recommended during pregnancy*. It is recommended for labour as it aids endurance and is an effective pain relief. It is renowned for relieving anxiety and nervous tension. Jasmine can be helpful after the birth when used as an adjunct to other therapies in mild cases of postnatal depression and exhaustion.
- **Clary sage** is also a uterine tonic and is therefore *not recommended during pregnancy*. It is known to assist contractions and the management of pain. It is also very relaxing for the mother during the birth and can be of assistance if she is anxious and distressed.
- Jasmine and clary sage are the essential oils of choice for birth when used in combination with lavender, geranium, sandalwood, neroli and mandarin, either for massage or used as a compress. All these oils should be used in a 1 to 2 per cent dilution in a good quality base carrier oil such as cold-pressed almond, avocado or apricot kernel oil. Or simply add five drops of each to 50 ml of the carrier oil.

For a relaxing aromatherapy massage during pregnancy create a warm and peaceful atmosphere with some favourite music and candles, or use the oils in a bath for complete relaxation.

During labour the position you choose might change as labour progresses and it is important that you and your birth support are both completely comfortable if you want to use massage. For example, if you are on the hands and knees or resting in the Child Pose, your birth support could sit on a low stool behind you, or beside you, to massage your lower back and sides. For abdominal massage, if you are on the floor or in bed they can sit behind you, supported by cushions as you lean against them. And while not always necessary, it is recommended that they remove any rings as these can be rough on your skin. Likewise, you might be inclined to grip your birth support's hands tightly during contractions, so it is advisable for both of you to take off your rings before the event, because rings can become very painful in this situation.

There is no set procedure with this type of massage—it's more about what is enjoyable at the time than technique. The degree of pressure is dependent on the area being massaged and what is needed most at the time. This can be a firm strong touch on the lower back, hips, shoulders and even the inner thighs, whereas massage on the face, neck and abdomen is always light and soft. Always let your birth support know if you would like them to change their technique or if you need to change position.

The scalp is a great place to start. Using firm finger pressure your birth support can massage slowly over the whole area, not forgetting the base of the skull where tension can build up, and continuing into the muscles of the neck, upper back and shoulders. Gentle massage the temples and forehead and across the eyebrow line from the eyebrow centre outwards towards the temples, either in small circles or long slow movements. You might prefer your face to be stroked slowly and softly for a very peaceful, dreamy result.

The shoulders and upper back can be massaged separately for a deep relaxing massage and to relieve upper body tension or as part of a full back massage.

A firm massage over the hips and lower back will relieve lower back pain by working into the muscles as if kneading bread. Remember always to avoid massaging on the spine itself. A light tickling in the centre of the lower back, between the hips in the area of the sacroiliac joint, gives a deep, relaxing effect even though the touch is so light.

If you are lying on your side your birth support can massage your back, your head and abdomen. Massage over the abdomen is very soothing and some women have found it particularly helpful during transition. It is best done in a slow circular movement that flows from the top of abdomen to the base of the belly, at the top of the pubic bone. This can also including the sides of the body and the waist. Keep the hands on the body moving slowly and constantly so that one hand follows the other for a continuous flowing motion.

Most people enjoy having their feet massaged and during labour a gentle foot massage can have a very relaxing effect on the whole body. Remember to apply the acupressure points here as well (ball of foot, between first and second toes).

During a contraction, firm pressure or a soft squeezing action can be applied to the inner thigh muscles from the groin to the knee to help relieve tension in these muscles and to draw the woman's awareness down into her body and to be less in her mind.

Endorphin-releasing Massage

This is a very gentle massage technique with the lightest touch which helps to create an immediate calmness in the mind and a sense of deep relaxation in the body. This lovely technique helps you to go into the most relaxed state possible, a so-called hypnotic state encouraging you to be relaxed and alert at the same time. Being calm and mindful go hand in hand with feelings of empowerment and trust, so when you're relaxed a steady confidence and inner strength are also present.

There are a number of ways to do this softer massage technique, which is often part of hypnobirthing. The birth support can place their hands on your shoulders and very slowly, with the lightest possible

touch, move their hands down your back to the base of the spine, or crossing the hands past each other as they move down the back—from left to right in a weaving movement. Or they can start with their hands on the crown of your head and slowly bring them all the way down your back.

This slow, soft fingertip pressure also feels wonderful down the side of the face, on the ear lobes and from the back of the neck towards the shoulders or down the insides of the arms—or really anywhere that the nerves are most sensitive to touch. It seems to be most effective when the movement is from the top to the bottom— that is, from the temple to the throat, or from the upper arm, especially down the inner arm towards to the fingertips. The movement is gentle and as soft as possible, and always very slow.

Practise these techniques with your birth support before the onset of labour so you become familiar with them. Your body will respond quickly by relaxing easily and the atmosphere of your mind will quieten and soften. Try repeating an appropriate word or affirmation as the fingertips lightly touch the body, or ask your birth support to do it as a way of carrying that awareness through the soft touch. Ask your birth support to do this during labour—for example … *open … relax … breathe out … I am birthing my baby easily and gently …* When the touch is moving from the top of the body downwards it encourages the mind to be drawn down

into the body, so that you are not so much in your thoughts, and your mind is with your baby in your womb, mentally and spiritually together as you progress through this extraordinary time.

Herbal Medicines

- **Raspberry leaf** is probably the most useful herb to consider during pregnancy as it is a uterine tonic. It is used by many women from the third trimester as a tea or in capsules, although some herbalists suggest using it before then. It has a toning effect on the uterine muscles and is useful after the birth for the same reason.

- For digestive upsets use **peppermint**, **spearmint** and a little **chamomile** as tea.

- **Nettle** tea is high in iron and is a wonderful tonic for pregnancy and good for kidney function.

- **Dandelion root** 'coffee' is a great alternative to regular coffee and is very good for liver and kidney function,

---

Caution: While many herbs are safe to use during pregnancy, many others are not. Herbal medicines should always be dispensed by a qualified naturopath or herbalist. If you choose to use herbal medicines during your pregnancy remember to inform your medical professionals.

remembering to always take it in moderation due to its diuretic affect.

- If you are anxious either before the birth or later on **skullcap**, **passionflower** and **lime flowers** as teas all have a calming, relaxing effect on the emotions.
- **St John's wort** is widely used for the treatment of mild anxiety and depression and is valuable for those reasons during pregnancy and after the birth. It is *not recommended after the birth* if you are taking the contraceptive pill, as it will interfere with the effectiveness of the pill.

While other herbals are also safe during pregnancy for other situations, I feel these are the ones to consider specifically for pregnancy and in preparation for birth. A herbal birth preparation mix for use in the last weeks of pregnancy can be made up by a naturopath or herbalist. This can be taken in conjunction with the Bach Flower remedies as a gentle way to bring about balance in the body and the mind.

Bach Flower and Bush Flower Remedies

The English Bach Flower and Australian Bush Flower remedies have special relevance for pregnancy, and especially for labour, because of their subtle yet profound abilities to balance and calm the emotions. For the most beneficial results consult a qualified practitioner rather then choosing a remedy yourself. The flower essences work on the emotional body and are best made up to suit your personal needs at a specific time and as your emotions change during pregnancy.

These remedies are safe to use during times of mental and emotional stress, indecision and confusion. It is important to point out that they will not fix or solve an emotional problem or issue, but they do seem to soften the heightened emotions associated with the issue. Often when we relax a little and our energy changes around a problem we are able to see it from a different perspective, and solutions can more easily be found.

The flower remedies are a non-invasive way of managing the emotional changes that occur during pregnancy. During labour they will gently relax you, easing your mind and emotions so you are able to stay with what is happening rather than becoming confused, fearful or disorientated. They are also very suitable after the birth, gently helping you move through the massive hormonal and emotional changes that naturally occur, and are especially helpful if you are having a difficult time with the after-birth 'blues'. I suggest having them in water which you can sip on during the day. If a more severe depression occurs after the birth, the flower remedies can be used in conjunction with other therapies and professional counselling. Remember, they will not resolve a problem on their own.

The remedies will also come to the 'rescue' if you are emotionally troubled while breast-feeding, as your frame of mind will influence your body's chemistry and therefore affect your breast milk. Even if you are not breast-feeding, your baby will instinctively know when you are upset and these remedies are good to have on hand. Under professional supervision they are safe and very effective to use in minute doses for your baby too.

Water Birth

Water is a beautiful medium to labour in, and to birth your baby. More and more women are choosing to use water during this time as it is gentle, soothing and deeply relaxing. Women who birth their babies at home very often do so in a birthing pool and many hospitals and birthing centres have a birth pool available. Sometimes a woman will spend part of her labour in the water and birth on 'land', others birth their babies in the water. It is considered a safe alternative to regular birthing under the supervision of professionals who are skilled in this birth choice. Water birth has many advantages worth considering.

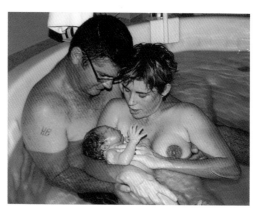

Janet Balaskas, in her wonderful *Water Birth Book*, lists the benefits of spending time in water during labour and birthing in water:

- Increases privacy.
- Provides significant pain relief.
- Reduces the need for drugs and interventions.
- Encourages a woman's sense of control in labour.
- Facilitates mobility and enables the woman to adopt optimal positions for an active birth.
- Speeds up labour.
- Promotes relaxation and conserves energy.
- Helps to reduce tears.
- Is rated highly by mothers and midwives.

- Encourages an easier birth for the mother and is gentler welcome for the baby (page 73).

Being in a warm bath is a wonderful way to relieve stress and physical discomfort. During labour being in a pool of warm water helps a woman to relax more easily, to open to childbirth, while her contractions are cushioned by the water. It also helps the perineum and cervix to relax and is especially valuable if she is tense and not dilating well, a situation which often improves once she moves into the water.

Some women feel safe in the smaller space of the birth pool. The birth support can be in the pool with her, making for skin to skin contact, a very intimate way to share the experience. They can hold and support her body if she is floating in a semi seated position. In most of the positions she is likely to use, massage can still be applied. Squatting is often too difficult to maintain for long on 'land', but in the water it can be managed more easily.

Deb Biffin's thoughts (see box below) about water birth are so beautiful and encouraging to all pregnant women, not only because of her wonderful experiences but also because her approach to childbirth is inspirational and embraces all the principles I have endeavoured to bring forth in this book. Her story is an example of how childbirth can be a positive and empowering journey from every perspective—physically, emotionally and especially spiritually—and that it can definitely be one of life's most incredible and satisfying journeys.

I believe water is the cradle of life, so to me, there was never a question that I wanted to labour and birth my babies in water. I have three children and all are water babies. I am currently pregnant again with my fourth child and plan to again birth in water.

Water offers so much more than just pain relief, it is peaceful and calm and totally envelops you with its warm, safe feeling. Labouring and birthing in water was emotionally and spiritually peaceful and gentle for my babies and for me too. Being in the water relaxed my body which then made it easier to stay 'in tune' with my body and my baby … to work with my body and to make my baby's journey easier, quicker, less stressful and ultimately more peaceful.

The birth of our third child, Tyler, was beautiful, almost beyond words. It was the first time my husband Steve, had entered the water with me. He helped me to float when I wanted to and was

my 'anchor' when I needed physical support in the weightless environment of water. We hummed together and just totally embraced the moment. As I hummed and gently pushed Tyler's head out, Steve's hand was there to help guide him. I then pushed out the rest of his little body and both Steve and I floated him to my chest, and welcomed him into the world. Our son was born. He was calm, relaxed and peaceful, just as his sisters were when they had entered the world in water too. No screaming or crying. He was welcomed into a safe and familiar environment—water—a mirror of my womb which had been his home for the past nine months. I am filled with elation when I think of the births of my three children. I believe giving birth is the most liberating and empowering event I will ever experience. I love water birth. I love giving birth. I love being a woman.

Art Therapy

The idea of using art therapy during pregnancy was brought to my attention in the wonderful book *Birthing from Within*, by Pam England and Rob Horowitz. Art therapy is a very interesting concept and a valuable tool to use during pregnancy for a number of reasons, as well as at other times not related to birth. Briefly, I have found it of great value as another way to access feelings, to identify emotions that need to be resolved and removed before the birth, to dissolve negative thoughts around the birthing process, and to move the awareness from pregnancy to life after birth. It is especially valuable if a previous experience, to do with pregnancy and birth, or some other time in life, has left an imprint of fear and self-doubt in the consciousness. I have used in it private consultation and in my birth preparation workshops, and when women come with their birth support, who really seem to enjoy this too. It is a gentle and intuitive way to look at your beliefs, conscious and unconscious, those that are positive and the ones that might be limiting you in some way. It enables you to get in touch with the hard-to-look-at feelings and accompanying negative emotions, and express them in a creative, fun and therapeutic way.

Art is also about bringing the most cherished feelings to life in a creative and sensitive way. Some women become interested in art for the first time during pregnancy and draw to help them with their own transformational journey. They find art is a way to honour themselves during this brief time and to put in a creative way their innermost feelings. It is also very helpful to shift the focus from pregnancy to the reality of birth, and life after birth.

I ask women to do three drawings: one of themselves now, one of the birth and the atmosphere they envisage and are hoping for, and one when they are at home with their new baby, their new family. I also encourage them to write empowering words or affirmations that come to mind as they draw, which many women have used during birth. Some women so enjoyed and benefited from the process that they had their drawings with them during labour; others have kept their drawings as part of their journey in pregnancy and childbirth, from one aspect of being a woman to another. One father was so impressed with the drawing of his new family, including the dog, the pool and the Lilo, that he intended to have it screen-printed on a T-shirt and wear it to the birth! *Birthing from Within* is an exceptional book and I recommend it to anyone who is having children or working with pregnancy and childbirth.

Hypnobirthing

The feeling experienced in hypnosis is very similar to what you feel in deep relaxation, or yoga nidra. The principles are the same, and both take you to a place in your mind where you are conscious, but have shifted into a deeper level of calm and peace. They both give benefits for dealing with pain and in managing anxiety and stress better and are both relevant in preparation for birth. When the hypnobirthing practices are used in conjunction with yoga breathing and visualisations you have a truly valuable combination of skills to refer to as you move through the birthing process. The breathing exercises, especially ujjayi breathing and humming, take you into a hypnotic type of space and encourage you to stay there, and move back into it if you become distracted or lose that calm feeling.

Many aspects of hypnosis for birth involve your birth support, who can help you to relax into a deep, calm state of mind, as well as the applying soft endorphin-releasing massage and touch techniques.

The Candle Meditation

Although it is not permitted to have a lit candle in hospital you might find the candle meditation valuable in the early stages of labour when you are still at home. If you are having your baby at home of course there are no restrictions on what you choose to do.

If you are able to stay at home in pre-labour and your waters have not yet broken, you can spend some time soaking in a warm bath with the essential oils recommended for birth and the candle flame in a position that is easy for you to see. With the atmosphere created, you can relax in the warm water and be calmed by the aromas while gazing at the brightest point of the flame. You might like to have your favourite music or chanting playing in the background to enhance the mood. This might seem a bit extreme when you are trying to cope with early contractions, but I have known women who have done exactly this, finding it a wonderful way to stay calm and prepare for the more active part of labour. After the birth the candle meditation creates a lovely ambience to relax and feed your new baby.

Sometimes a woman in the early moments of labour during a class has

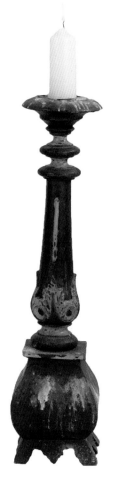

chosen to stay in that calm supportive environment as her contractions progressed. Two such occasions come to mind, once when we were doing the candle meditation and another time when we were using ujjayi breathing for a deep meditation. The two women commented later how much they enjoyed being with the class and how this reflective time helped them stay calm and centred. They were able to use this opportunity in the quiet of the meditation to prepare mentally and emotionally for the more active part of labour. This enabled them to stay relaxed and very aware of what was happening in their body and to reflect on the absolute wonder of this amazing time. Being in a meditative state as the contractions gently came and went gave them the opportunity to breathe with each surge, to be totally centred and focused and to be there with their baby. It was a very special time for all of us, a rare privilege to be witness to this private, sacred moment in the life of these women, to be part of the precious moments of a new life unfolding. We were able to support them just by being there with thoughts of love for the women and welcome to their baby. These times embraced the miracle of life and the wonder of being a woman and acknowledged the ever-present bond between women, and the very special understanding all birthing women and mothers share. It was a great joy to share in these very rare and exquisite times and

I am ever grateful that I have been able to provide the space for women to connect in this beautiful way, to truly honour the feminine and life in utero.

Music

Some women find it comforting to have a favourite piece of music or sacred chant playing in the background during labour to soothe and relax them. During pregnancy spend some time listening to your favourite music, especially if it has a relaxing and calming influence so it can be used for the same effects during labour.

Crystals

Crystals are a wonder of our natural world and are beautiful whether in their original state or made into fine jewellery. They have been used throughout history in ceremony and as a sign of wealth and social standing while their therapeutic value is becoming more accepted

Pregnant women often become drawn to the beauty of crystals for their natural beauty and colour. The same qualities relate to the colour of crystals as to the colours in colour healing and visualisation (see page 177).

A number of crystals are considered appropriate for pregnancy and birthing, although it is very much a personal choice. Some women like to have a small selection of different stones with them during the birth, especially when they are aware of their qualities and energies.

Clear or white stones are associated

with mental clarity and wisdom. During pregnancy moonstone is the best choice. In India it is considered excellent for women of all ages, bringing balance to their emotions. It is used to ease PMS and has significant benefits where there are fluctuations in mood and emotions. Moonstone is associated with water, and as there is a tendency for increased fluid retention during pregnancy and for more emotional sensitivity, it is a natural choice. Pearls, like moonstone associated with the emotions and water, are also have special relevance during pregnancy, being feminine in nature and resembling the luminous quality of the moon.

Black or darker stones, including black tourmaline, hematite and variations of obsidian, are very relevant, as they are being about grounded and focused, connected to the earth and your physical self. Where there is restlessness due to mental stress and confusion they encourage stability and are valuable for inner reflection or when there is a need to internalise more. I recommend hematite as it calms and relaxes the mind and is said to have a positive influence on iron levels in the blood.

The beautiful rose quartz is associated with calming the emotions and bringing peacefulness to the heart, and is a favourite during pregnancy. Red coral, ruby and garnet have similar qualities while ruby is also good for circulation on a physical level, and gives courage and relief from doubt in the emotions.

Green stones such as jade and aventurine help us connect to nature and the earth and to feel more centred in the physical body. Green crystals help to soothe the emotions and where the breath is restricted they encourage deeper breathing.

Dark blue stones such as lapis lazuli and sodalite increase intuition and heighten spiritual awareness and can bring a deep peacefulness in the mind. During pregnancy women are often drawn to the beauty of lapis, which can help you access greater wisdom from within yourself and to trust your insights.

Amethyst is a favourite with many women for the gentle qualities attributed to it and the way it calms the mind during times of stress. Even if you are relaxed and calm during pregnancy and birth, amethyst will bring greater peace and tranquillity.

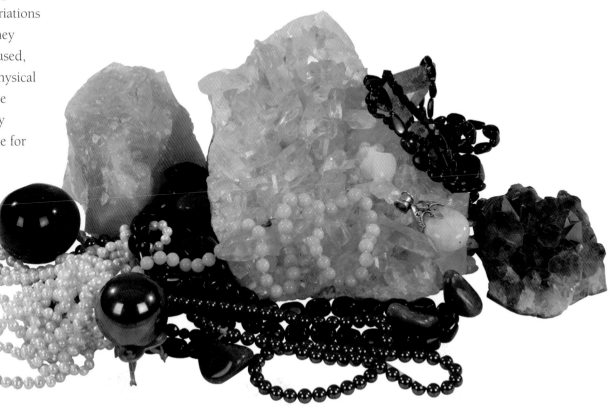

CHAPTER 18

THE ROLE OF YOUR BIRTH SUPPORTS

I have spoken often of the value of birth supports, but not said much about what they do.

The medical team present at the time of your labour are your primary birth support, as they have the expertise and knowledge to assist you and your baby. Their presence makes you feel safe and confident and free to focus your attention on the birth.

Your family and friends are your other birth support and are there to share this very special and personal experience, and to give you encouragement and love. Their role is very important and you chose them because they know you intimately, they understand you, they love you and your baby and are there to support you in the best way they can.

For these reasons it is important for your birth support to be as well informed as possible about what to expect and

what could occur. Most of these topics are discussed in detail at the hospital antenatal classes that are part of your pregnancy care. Most birth units are very willing for you to bring things you feel might be useful during the birth that are not medical in nature. This might include your favourite music, aromatherapy and massage oils, herbal and homeopathic remedies, a bean bag if it's not part of the regular equipment, and even the stool you have been using for yoga.

If you are intending to use some of the breathing and relaxation techniques you have learnt during labour, it is important for your birth support to be familiar with them too, so they can help you follow them. This also applies to having an understanding of the positions that can be used, aromatherapy massage, visualisations and hypnobirthing relaxation practices. Even though you might use only a few of these things,

having someone there who is aware of them can help you to stay calm and relaxed, and give you encouragement. Their active involvement will make an enormous difference to you and how you manage the challenges that might present themselves as labour progresses.

Always have someone with you or close by rather than being left alone, and try to let them know how you are feeling even when the going gets tough. Often this is enough encouragement for you to stay positive and to surrender to the flow of labour.

Some women don't move much during labour, preferring to find a comfortable position and stay in it, some don't want to talk or even open their eyes—all of this is normal. Becoming still in the body and being quiet and more internalised is still being active in the birth—active in your focus, where your thoughts are taking you, and breathing consciously, just not active in your body. It is also worth knowing that not all women want to be touched during labour so that you and your birth support don't get upset if this happens to you. Feeling like this may make it easier to concentrate on the feelings in your body and stay connected to your baby.

Here are some suggestions for all birth supports, not just the father of the baby. Not all will be suitable in your situation but all are worth consideration. It is also worthwhile reading part IV, Complementary therapies.

Encourage the birthing mother:

※ To relax as much as possible between each contraction, to rest and recover and to prepare for the next one, body, mind and spirit.

※ To have a positive attitude about the contractions, to remember that they are a celebration and each one brings her closer to the birth of her baby.

※ To centre her mind with the various breathing exercises, especially ujjayi breathing, humming and relaxed conscious breathing. Remind her of the potential in each and every breath.

※ To use her affirmations and any other visualisations that she especially likes.

※ Remind her to trust in herself, to surrender to the feelings in her body and to go with the phenomenal power

of labour, to keep her mouth open and soft with the jaw relaxed and the teeth apart, of the association between the cervix and relaxation throughout the pelvic floor.

※ Tell her throughout how wonderful she is, that she is doing really well, and if you are her partner use the private, intimate way of speaking that you both understand. She will respond to your voice and especially the tone of your voice. At transition you might tell her that the birth is very close now, if that feels appropriate. Your role is to be attentive and calm, always using encouraging, positive language with short simple phrases: relax now ... *breathe ... you're doing really well ...open and relax ... well done ...*

※ Breathe with her, talk to her, hum with her and to the baby. Keep eye contact if that feels appropriate.

※ Offer her sips of cool liquids and ice. Keep her warm but not hot.

※ Focus with her on the cervix becoming soft and open in preparation for birth, remind her of the flower meditation and what it represents. Remind her to relax the perineum and pelvic floor muscles, to open softly and gently as she dilates. When you are both concentrating on the same thing the influence is much more powerful

and focused. This shared meditation encourages her to open and relax more readily and to stay in touch with what is actually happening.

※ The baby as well as the mother is involved in the birthing process, so remind her to reconnect with her baby as often as possible with words of love and welcome, again you can both be involved.

※ During the second stage help her to focus her energy down into the birth canal, visualising her body opening to welcome her baby, and to breathe consciously as she knows. Encourage deep relaxation, using the mind with the breath to surrender to the power of the surges, to let go, to open her body to birth her baby. This will enable her to centre and be more in control, thereby preventing over-straining and exhaustion. Let her know she is surrounded in love, and that her baby is loved and welcome.

※ Use the endorphin-releasing massage (page 154) and soft touch techniques to take her into a deep relaxed state. Use encouraging words or phrases as you do this.

※ Help her find a comfortable resting position, re-arrange the cushions, bean bag and maybe apply massage if requested.

✳ Apply a warm cloth to the perineum to encourage relaxation.

✳ Use acupressure points to relieve pain during a contraction. These include firm finger pressure on the centre of the ball of the foot, or between the first and second toes on the soft fleshy pad of the foot. Another point is at the base of the thumb joint on the front of the hand, where the crease ends between the thumb and the first finger. This point is stimulating to the uterus and is best not used if she is being induced. Other points on the lower back and hips can be reached with deep massage.

✳ Flower remedies can be offered throughout labour.

✳ The essential oil clary sage can be added to a warm damp cloth, approximately five drops, and be placed on her abdomen or for her to inhale. Other essential oils recommended for labour can be used instead or as well (see page 153).

✳ Cool her face with a flannel—this can also have a few drops of essential oil on it. To help her relax use lavender, neroli or geranium; to give her courage use sandalwood and rosewood; to clear her mind use mandarin and orange. Hypericum is a wonderful non-aromatic oil to relieve nerve pain and can be massaged into the lower back and sacrum area. Play music or other sound CDs she has chosen if appropriate.

✳ And don't forget the camera.

✳ After the birth, make sure she is warm and comfortable because the shock of birthing can make her cold and shivering. Some women are starving by now, and some favourite light snacks might be acceptable. A warm broth is very nourishing and helps to restore energy, for example, barley and vegetables or a light chicken broth. Or you might prefer to celebrate with a vintage champagne.

Write the important points down so you have a record of them with you when labour begins. Remember the birthing experience can be unnerving and stressful for you too, especially if she is in pain and you don't know what to do to take the pain away. If you are a man, although it is in your nature to want to fix things and make everything better, in this case take pain and discomfort away, remember that your *presence* is what she needs and often all she needs to help her relax.

If the labour is long, make sure you keep up your own fluids and nourishment so that your energies are not depleted. She will be needing you for the duration and you will want to be there to support her, and to be there at the moment of birth.

Sheila Kitzinger, in *The New Pregnancy and Childbirth*, speaks about the importance of the role of the birth support person:

When you are with a woman in childbirth, you share with her a journey into the unknown. Giving support during labour needs vigilance, skill, patience, an understanding of that particular woman—her rhythms, her response to stress—an awareness of what she is thinking and how she is feeling in each moment, and your complete commitment to this task. Sometimes it demands endurance and courage. It can be hard, exhausting work. But yours, too, is the excitement, the deep satisfaction and joy when a child is born (page 276).

CHAPTER 19

SKILLS FOR BIRTH: TRUST. SURRENDER. ACCEPT

Trust in yourself, totally, as woman and as a mother, trust in your body, your birth support and your medical team. Surrender to the amazing energy of birth, with no resistance, and relinquish any attempt at control over the unpredictable, give over to it in your mind, in your body and in your soul. Accept that labour is a mystery, and mystical. Discover your inner strength, tap into your innate feminine knowing, and have the courage to completely go with the circumstances that present on the birthday of your baby. You are unique, as is your labour and your baby's birth experience. Be filled with grace and love. Love yourself and love your baby, feel the love surrounding you both. Embrace this beautiful, extraordinary moment in your life as a woman, as a mother, and the new soul that is your baby. Realise the miracle of life and its absolute preciousness. Relax and allow your intuition, your woman's inner knowing and wisdom to guide you.

When you are focused and centred in yourself—with the knowledge that you have prepared for this time mentally, emotionally and physically—you will have the self-trust, inner strength and confidence to approach labour with a clear mind and a positive attitude. You will be able to utilise all your physical strength and mental energies to be actively involved in the different stages of the birthing process with a one pointed awareness and sense of purpose. Even if things don't go exactly as planned your attitude, and the various skills you have learnt through yoga, will still prove to be of great benefit and support to you.

By now you will be familiar with most of the suggestions here. The most important consideration is that on this birthday of your baby, you are both safe and well. This is undoubtedly one of the most precious moments in your life, to be fully embraced and enjoyed. But whatever happens on the day, always trust in your inherent feminine wisdom and move with the birthing process consciously and with acceptance, acknowledging that there are times in life that are unpredictable. Even if the birth is very different from what you had always hoped for you have still nurtured your baby throughout pregnancy, and will continue to once your baby is born.

I am confident that if you have spent even a short time learning, practising and gaining an understanding of the skills recommended in this book you will remember to use some of them, at some point, even if only at the onset of labour or for a short time.

You may not use them all the time but I believe you will intuitively use those that are the most suitable at the time, especially those that gave you the most benefit during pregnancy. This is the case whether it is a natural vaginal birth, a vaginal birth with medical intervention or a caesarean. Many women have used these skills as preparation where a caesarean delivery is required, or during the procedure as a way of remaining as calm and relaxed as possible. In all these situations, the more centred and positive you are the better it will be for you and your baby and those supporting you, including your medical team. When you are calm and coping well, you are also together and strong, better guided from your own inner knowing and therefore more confident. The atmosphere in your mind and in your womb is then relaxed and peaceful, a feeling which will flow over those supporting you.

Some women assume that when the time comes to use the breathing and visualisation techniques to assist them during labour, their skills will 'go out the window'. Although this does happen sometimes, the majority of women do use these skills at some point, to their great benefit, simply because they have faith in their knowledge and belief in the practices. They are able to trust in themselves completely and in those supporting them, to surrender to the unknowns of the birthing process and to accept whatever this day brings with it. Trust. Surrender. Accept.

When you come to know and trust your own source of inner strength from deep within your feminine nature, it will be there for you 'on call', not only during labour and birth but when you encounter challenges along life's unpredictable path. Embrace a willingness to become one with the energy of birthing, rather than trying to control the process. Birth is a very positive experience for many women and can be for you also. When birth is approached with acceptance and a sense of what is real it brings with it a quiet confidence you will enjoy for many years to come.

A Birth Plan

Labour cannot really be planned, rarely goes to schedule and definitely cannot be controlled. Because of this it is better to prepare yourself with what you feel you can use confidently during the birth journey rather than attempting to stick to a rigid plan. A birth plan that is flexible is always worthwhile as it enables you and your birth support to concentrate your attention on the birth of a new precious soul. A simple, realistic plan gives you and your birth support the opportunity to talk about what feels acceptable and comfortable, and what you have strong feelings against. Talking it through and writing down a birth plan brings more awareness of what you might encounter on the day and how you might best cope. The less rigid and more real it is, the better prepared you will be.

Sometimes a woman will be overwhelmed with understandable disappointment when a natural birth didn't eventuate or she had to rely on analgesics instead of managing a drug-free birth. If left unresolved, disappointment can lead to bonding and feeding problems and detachment from their beautiful, healthy baby. It can remain problematic long after the birth, resulting in depression, low self-esteem and lack of confidence, especially when she becomes pregnant again and is nearing the time of birth. This highlights the fact that it's crucial to know where your focus is and what is most important during birth.

The birth of your baby is one of life's most awe-inspiring moments. It is the incredible time you have long waited for, when you finally meet each other, mother and child. And while you want the journey to be natural, and as calm and peaceful as possible, it is your attitude and willingness to surrender that could make all the difference between it being a positive and empowering experience, or one that is fraught with disappointment.

Breathing for Birth

Every breath you take gives you energy and prana.

The breath gives life and sustains life. It is powerful yet gentle.

The incoming breath is always nourishing and replenishing for your mind, your body and your soul.

The outgoing breath is always about release and relaxation, it is powerful and cleansing.

When you breathe consciously it is empowering and centring, every breath has unlimited potential. Breathing consciously keeps you present and awake.

Breath awareness is pure meditation. It keeps you mindful of the preciousness and transient nature of each and every moment.

Breath awareness is internalising and connects you to your feminine wisdom and inner strength, and opens you to greater insight and intuition. It connects you to your baby in your womb.

Mindfulness of the breath encourages you to feel calm and positive. It makes you feel steady and balanced. It gives you confidence and courage and makes you feel strong in yourself.

Breath awareness helps you to surrender to the process of birth, to accept, to trust.

All these ideas come to mind in thinking about birth and what yoga breathing can bring to birthing your baby. There is really no correct way to breathe during labour, only that you must breathe efficiently and consciously. It is the opinion of many who assist women through labour that it is best to leave it up to the woman. Although there is truth in that, most women I meet want to know how to breathe during labour and childbirth. Labour happens to you but how you breathe will greatly influence how you manage what labour brings with it.

A woman who has learnt some of the yoga breathing techniques and how to breathe correctly is able to steady and calm her mind, relax herself and work with the energy of birthing. She will approach labour and progress through the contractions with greater confidence and strength from within herself.

I am not suggesting that if yoga breathing or some form of meditation is not followed during pregnancy that the birth experience won't be fulfilling, but rather that these skills give women something to tap into, to trust in and use actively not only during labour but for the rest of their lives.

The techniques recommended here are only guidelines, based on what women have been using with great benefit since I began teaching pregnancy yoga. You might use some of the breathing exercises recommended, or simply bring your awareness to the natural breath and use that as a guide to move from one contraction to the next. The most important point to remember is to breathe and to breathe well, whether that is deep breathing, humming or just the quiet breath—and to be conscious of the potential in the breath and how it can most help you.

The energy of labour can sometimes take a woman by surprise and carry her far beyond what feels familiar and safe, it can be overwhelming and a little frightening. But it can also be a very positive and powerful experience. Prepare yourself for labour by being familiar with your favourite breathing exercises and visualisation techniques. Always choose the practices that gave you the most benefits during pregnancy as they are the ones that will give you the best opportunity to work deeply with your body and the amazing energy of birth. It is not unusual for women to feel that an unknown 'greater' part of themselves emerges during labour where they come to know and experience the wonder and miracle of giving birth—and of life itself. By utilising your breath, the energy within it and its extraordinary potential, you have the ability to be completely aware during labour, to stay clearly focused in the present and to call on your own natural wisdom. You will then move through the birthing process confidently and calmly rather than feeling fear and tension and struggling against what the day brings. The principle is the same as having your bag packed ready for hospital, only with these skills and suggestions you are well prepared mentally and spiritually with some valuable resources ready to use during labour.

When practising the breathing exercises, always keep in mind that the incoming breath supplies you with prana and all that you need to maintain balance and harmony in your body, mind and spirit. The outgoing breath is there to release tension, anxiety and stress and importantly to help you relax. Being the witness and observer of your natural breath as it moves gently in and out of your body is the key to staying relaxed and centred, to be as one with yourself and to have your attention firmly in the present.

The breathing techniques can be used with the surge of a contraction, during a contraction and while resting. Having the thought in mind that every contraction is a celebration is often very helpful—each contraction is one less that you will ever have, and brings you and your baby ever closer to meeting each other.

Ujjayi Pranayama

All the breathing practices have many benefits for labour but ujjayi pranayama is probably the most important and valuable technique, and is used consistently with positive results. It can be used in any of its many variations—including as a gentle meditative breath during a contraction or between contractions to hold you in a deep, relaxed, hypnotic state. The throat breathing can be done on its own or in conjunction with deep breathing, or with the tongue resting against the soft palate and the mouth slightly open. It is especially good if you lose concentration or become restless, particularly as you approach transition where you might begin to feel scattered and vague. One or two conscious throat breaths will very quickly take you back into a deeply relaxed space where you are quiet and centred again, especially when done in conjunction with your affirmations or a single empowering word.

A client of mine (I'll call her Shannon) went into labour six weeks early and was distressed and very frightened by her unexpected contractions. By coincidence I was supporting a friend in her labour at the same hospital on that day. Shannon was given an epidural and hooked up to a monitor. Although she couldn't feel the contractions it was clear from the monitor that her baby was becoming more distressed with each one. The medical staff said that if her baby continued to be distressed, she was most likely going to need a caesarean. Shannon had always enjoyed the ujjayi breathing and gained a lot of benefit from it, so I suggested she use that to help her relax and hopefully calm her baby. It was extraordinary to witness how quickly she relaxed, and because of that her baby's heart rate became more regular, and in the end there was no need for a caesarean. Everyone, including the medical staff, was obviously relieved, but also very impressed at the remarkable effect the breathing had on Shannon and her unborn baby. Because we could see the reading on the monitor changing as she continued with ujjayi breathing, there was technical evidence to validate the calming response in her, and on her baby.

The Cooling Breath

The Cooling Breath is very centring and easy to focus on due to the sensation of cool air on your tongue. It can be done with deep breathing or with the natural breath. When practising it I suggest you visualise a beautiful place in nature, somewhere you have been or a place you would love to visit, and 'draw' the feeling of that place into your mind as the breath comes into your body. The mind responds very well to pleasant thoughts and images and this concept will increase the effectiveness of the breath. It is also helpful to visualise a healing colour being drawn in with the breath, to enhance the feelings most needed at the time.

In conjunction with these visualisations focus on a word or a brief statement that is positive and makes you feel confident, and repeat it to yourself as you inhale. This will keep your attention firmly on what is nourishing and empowering and help you to be more in the present moment. These techniques encourage you to stay relaxed and strong and can be used from pre-labour to after the birth.

Abdominal Breathing

Abdominal breathing is very important for labour and can be used with the mouth either open or closed, and with the other techniques recommended here. It can be done continuously, and its value comes from having a complete focus and awareness on the abdominal area—the part of your body where you are feeling the contractions. Any strong emotions will be felt in the abdomen and the more relaxed this area is during the birthing process the better you will feel. Breathing into this part of the body will help the muscles relax which means less discomfort. If you don't have enough oxygen coming into the body, the muscles are not being replenished and the contractions tend to be more intense.

Conscious abdominal breathing also means you can direct your attention to that part of the body, to be there with your baby in your womb, moment to moment. If you have a tendency to hold your breath or repeatedly take short, rapid breaths into the upper chest, hyperventilation can result. This is very unsettling and makes you feel dizzy, light-headed, disorientated and less together, as well as producing tingling in the extremities. Relaxed abdominal breathing will stabilise your breathing quickly so you can again work consciously with your body as labour progresses.

Deep Yoga Breathing

Deep Yoga Breathing is an extremely valuable exercise to use throughout labour, especially when you remain conscious of the potential within each breath. The incoming breath will replenish your energy and nourish you in the most positive way, and help you to feel confident and empowered. The outgoing breath is about the release of tensions on all levels thereby helping you to relax deeply and to stay focused on yourself and your baby. Take a deep breath at the onset of a contraction to help you focus and to draw in the prana and energy you will need for the contraction. When the contraction has ended deeper breathing will equalise the breath in your body and help you to relax in preparation for the next one. However, I recommend taking only two or three deep breaths at a time. When you are breathing deeply, repeat a positive word or statement to help create the atmosphere that will most benefit you. Or you might like to visualise a strong feminine energy in the form of light or a particular colour filling your mind and body. Some women draw strength from bringing to mind a woman who has

inspired them, living or historical, a figure who inspires them and carries the symbol of birthing women and of the mother.

The Cleansing Breath

The Cleansing Breath is excellent for releasing tension and stress on all levels. As you exhale strongly through your mouth, imagine all tension and discomfort being blown out and away from your body and mind, leaving you relaxed and calm. When your mouth is open there is less tension in your face and scalp which helps you to feel open and relaxed to birthing your baby. Remember to think about the connection between your mouth being open, the perineum being relaxed and the cervix softening and opening to birth your baby. The cleansing breaths can also be done continuously with a quiet, natural breath—breathing in through the nose and softly out through the mouth. The emphasis is always on relaxing consciously with each outgoing breath.

The Humming Breath

The Humming Breath enables you to centre your mind and to tune in with your own unique healing sound. It is also thought to have an influence on releasing the natural endorphins in the body. Many women have used the Humming Breath during labour to help overcome pain, to stay focused in the present moment, and to increase their inner strength by adding the dimension of sound to their great effort. They found it extremely

powerful to hum through the more intense contractions in the later stages of labour, feeling and visualising the vibrations moving deeply into their womb.

It really helps to make some noise during labour and is a completely natural thing to do. The sound you make is probably one which you've never heard yourself make before, yet at the same time is both familiar and extremely potent. When the time comes to increase the energy and strength required for childbirth the sound often heard is deep, primordial and ancient. It is a unique sound, characteristic to all birthing women and connecting them to each other. The Humming Breath resembles this deep feminine sound and connects you with your inner self, where the sound is like ripples of healing vibrations that move through your body and deep into your womb. You and your baby will both feel this soft sensation and hear the healing sound at same time. The intensity of labour can cause a woman to become too involved with the noise in her head and distracted from her body. When you hum the vibrations are heard constructively in the chest and abdomen and focus your attention on your body and your baby.

The Humming Breath will compose and centre your mind, while connecting you with an extraordinary stillness and peace deep inside, so valuable during labour. When the contractions begin to intensify, focus your awareness inwards and inhale slowly, drawing in all the prana and energy you will need. This can be very effective if you imagine you are drawing this powerful energy in through the top of the head, through the crown chakra. Breathe out and hum deeply while concentrating your whole awareness on moving the energy from your mind down into your womb, to your baby and into the birth canal. As you breathe in, repeat a single empowering word, or a short positive statement which is then carried with the sound and vibration as you exhale to help you birth your baby gently and consciously

Deb Biffin wrote about humming during labour:

During the birth of Jessica I used the humming breath and it definitely helped me to stay focused and calm and to channel my energy in a positive way. I used it to visualise my baby moving down the birth canal and to hum the pain away. Humming during labour felt like I was communicating with my baby and because I had done it so regularly throughout my pregnancy the sound was familiar to my baby. Jessica is now 15 months and I have continued to use the humming to soothe her when she is upset or to calm her at bedtime. I believe it definitely contributed to me having a wonderful, positive and natural birth experience. P.S. I have since used it during the births of my other two children.

Steve Biffin's thoughts on humming:
I first learnt about humming when I attended a birth preparation class with Theresa with my wife Deb. I wasn't sure if humming was something I would feel comfortable doing but once Deb's contractions became stronger it felt natural for me to hum with her, and I think it definitely helped her manage the pain. It is quite natural for husbands/partners to feel a bit helpless during labour but humming with Deb really made me feel like I was contributing. I feel it helped us to bond and really share the birth experience. I would never have imagined that humming would have been such a positive and wonderful effect on our birth experience.

Suggestions for Labour

Labour and childbirth are a time to be completely absorbed in yourself, your baby and the process of childbirth. Remember you are not in labour alone but are there with your baby, so constantly communicate with your baby and imagine her moving easily through the birth canal. Placing your hands on your abdomen during this time will help you connect with your baby, who I am sure will feel the warmth of your touch and sense the softness of your thoughts. Ujjayi pranayama and humming are especially good for focusing inwards as you move through the labour together mother and child, as one.

In nature most animals instinctively look for a quiet, dark and safe place to birth their young, on their own and away from their own kind. This allows them to birth peacefully and privately away from external disturbances. It is also what women knowingly seek, being a wisdom innate in all women so they are free to bring their awareness inwards to birth consciously and intuitively.

Birth is a very private and intimate experience and you need to feel safe, loved and in an environment that supports you on all levels. The place you have chosen to birth your baby should be warm and airy and wherever possible with the lights dimmed a little to create a softer ambience and encourage you to internalise more, to be mindful of yourself. A quieter more private space will enable you to withdraw inwards to be completely absorbed in the birth of your baby. A peaceful atmosphere helps the natural flow of the birthing process and because you are calm and relaxed you body will respond by releasing the right hormones at the right time.

Pre-labour

Pre-labour is the early feelings most women experience before real labour is established and it can last for a few hours, and sometimes for days. It might feel like period pain or a dull ache in the lower back that can be there continuously or come and go. It can be felt as very mild, softer contractions that are erratic, sometimes 15 or more minutes apart, that are there one day and gone the next, and because of this can be very confusing for new mums and their birth support.

Pre-labour is often exhausting so it is important to spend as much time as possible resting and relaxing to preserve

WARNING: If the waters show any discolouration, this is due to the presence of meconium, your baby's first bowel movement, and indicates your baby is distressed, or has been. This can be dangerous and getting to hospital immediately is essential.

valuable energy for when you will need it the most. It is common for the bowels to empty in preparation for proper labour, to be nauseated, for the mucus plug to be released, called a 'show' (it can be slightly bloodstained), or for the waters to break. It is advisable to call your hospital or midwife when these symptoms occur.

Not all women experience pre-labour but it is an opportunity to practise your breathing and visualisations and some of the other skills recommended here. Pelvic rocking on your hands and knees or standing, the Child Pose resting over a bean bag, some easy modified squatting or standing squatting will provide comfort, especially if you are experiencing backache. Gentle rocking can also be done on an exercise ball. Aromatherapy massage and the flower essences will help you relax and rest during this time and homeopathic remedies may also be indicated.

Contractions (surges)

In both first and second stage labour, as a contraction begins focus and centre your mind, relax your body as much

as possible into the most comfortable position and steady your breathing. A full deep breath can be taken as you move into the contraction bringing with it courage and strength. Focus on the outgoing breath with your mouth open and your jaw relaxed, breathing away discomfort or pain and consciously opening your body for birth.

The time between contractions is nature's way of giving you the opportunity to turn your attention inwards, to focus on restoring your strength and to come to a place of steadiness again. Use this time to rest and relax completely, to recover from the last contraction, to prepare physically and emotionally for the next one and connect with your baby.

When a contraction finishes, relax in the most comfortable position, moving your awareness inwards, visualising the energy within your breath restoring and replenishing your whole being. Talk to your baby, affirm that you are both doing fine and are so close now to meeting each other. Maybe visualise yourself and your baby surrounded by a beautiful colour. Close your eyes and feel your breath moving deeply into your body as you meditate and focus on its healing power. Remember each contraction is a celebration, each one bringing you closer to meeting your baby.

The natural breath, ujjayi breathing and humming all bring about a sense of calm and inner peace and can be used in conjunction with some of your favourite

affirmations. You might bring to mind the powerful image of the flower unfolding its petals and opening to the world, just as your body is opening to birthing your baby. Imagine, and feel the cervix becoming softer and dilating or see a colour at the mouth of the womb. These are especially potent ways for your mind and body to work together for a beautiful and fulfilling birth experience.

If the contractions are close together you might completely forget about breathing, especially if you are in transition, which probably means the birth is not too far away. However, your preparation before transition will make a difference to how you cope with it. You might only have the awareness to take one or two deep replenishing breaths but remember it is all helpful.

If the contractions are not close together, alternate nostril breathing will restore balance and relax the nervous system. Slow deep cleansing breaths aid in releasing tension and are appropriately followed by deep cooling or yogic breaths. Or simply find comfort in following the natural breath and being mindful of that.

First Stage

The first stage of labour is when the contractions are more established and stronger, are closer together and progressively more intense. As you progress through this stage the cervix dilates from what it was in pre-labour to 7 or 8 centimetres. Your whole attention will be taken up with these strong sensations but the more relaxed and centred you are the better you will stay with what is happening. Remember to just focus on one contraction at a time.

Breathe intuitively with what your body is doing as it moves in and out of the contraction. Relax and be present so you can best use all your energies. Often it helps to breathe in through the nose and out through the mouth, with mouth and jaw relaxed, always focusing on breathing discomfort and pain away.

A common response to pain is to clench your teeth and tighten your jaw and facial muscles, which in turn causes the muscles in your scalp, neck and shoulders to be tight and tense—as if to move away from the pain, to be separate from it. But tightness in the upper body can mean there more tension in the abdomen and the pelvic floor muscles, giving you the odd sensation that your head and body are disconnected, that you are detached from what is really happening in your body. This results in more physical discomfort, and less ability to surrender and go with the process of birth. You need to be focused on what you are feeling in your abdomen, in your womb and with your baby.

Some women prefer to breathe a little faster as the contraction grows in intensity, breathing in unison with the sensations, but always breathing in and out evenly. Others find it more beneficial to breathe slowly and more deeply. The more relaxed you can stay the more likely you will know which is best for you and remember to be flexible in what you do.

Do not hold your breath, keep the breathing steady and fluid. Even when the contractions mount in intensity find a pace and rhythm and go with that. As the contraction reaches the peak breathe with it, never against it. Sometimes it is helpful to think about a contraction as a huge wave—as the contraction grows in intensity it is like coming to the crest of the wave, and as it lessens you are coming down the other side of it.

When the contraction begins to ease off, synchronise your breathing with the lessening intensity, and when it is over take another slow full breath, with the emphasis on relaxing and releasing tension. If your breathing is short and shallow, balance it again when the contraction finishes by taking one or two slow deep breaths. As you move into transition, continue to go with your body and breathe through that process, and especially what your midwife recommends.

Remember to relax after a contraction and continually affirm that you are one contraction closer to meeting your baby. Be positive with your progress and support yourself and your effort, and remember to talk to your baby as you move through this process together.

Transition

Transition is the end of the first stage and before you are in the second stage of labour where you will be actively pushing. The cervix during transition is dilated between 8 and 10 centimetres. This time can be very disorienting and women often feel out of it, frightened, emotional, irritable, exhausted, angry, sometimes abusive—especially to their partners!—and very restless. The pain felt at transition can be very intense and overwhelming. Many women say after the birth that at transition they had had more than enough and wanted pain relief, or that they wanted to go home and forget all about giving birth—better to come back another day! Transition is a very internalised part of labour and some women don't want to talk or be touched, just wanting to stay within themselves, while others want to be held and to feel safe and supported.

Your birth support may feel surprised and quite concerned by such hard-to-reach, changed behaviour, but it's natural and a sign that birth is closer. Some women find they have to make a very clear decision now, a definite choice of what direction to take—either to gather all their mental energies and move confidently and courageously through this phase, or to ask for analgesics. Pain relief is a personal choice, but at this point many women find their determination and strength diminished through sheer exhaustion and the enormous effort of labour.

During transition move if you need to, change position and be as comfortable as possible. The contractions can be all over the place, on top of each other, or even stop for a time. Suggestions for how to breathe are not really practical here, as you will do what is best for you or be guided by your midwife. Try to be relaxed and to remember that anxiety and fear inhibit the release of natural endorphins, the body's inbuilt mechanism to help relieve pain.

Surrender to the powerful energy of these moments. Trust in your feminine energies. Call on the symbol of birthing women and mothers through time, imagining the flower fully open. You may prefer the camera lens meditation and see your body open to the light inside your womb, to your baby. Remember you are giving birth not only to your baby's body, but to the soul within the body, the completely new and unique individual who has a life path of her own. Many women have said how helpful it was to shift their awareness to the precious soul their baby is within the body being born. Trust your body that it can birth your baby. Trust your intuition and your innate feminine knowing, feel confident, gather your strengths and surrender to the energy of birth. You and your baby are loved and supported. Imagine and feel your cervix reaching full dilation and your baby's head there in readiness to meet life outside your womb. Rest and relax as much as possible, stay calm and strong.

Second Stage

In the second stage of labour your cervix is fully dilated at 10 centimetres, when the pushing part of labour begins. Before you feel the overwhelming urge to push the contractions sometimes stop completely. If this happens use this time to rest and relax deeply, to restore your energies and prepare mentally and physically for this energetic phase. The birth of your baby is very close. Her head puts pressure on the pelvic floor muscles and the nerves in that part of the body, resulting in the desire to push. Known as Ferguson's reflex, this is a natural response and for many women is very empowering and energising. The hormone adrenaline is now naturally released to make you feel more awake and to give you the energy to actively birth your baby.

Sometimes your midwife will place her fingers on the perineum to guide you where to push effectively. Some women find it very helpful to have a mirror placed so that they can see what is happening as well as feel it. It helps at this time to relax the muscles of the pelvic floor so remember the breathing for the pelvic floor exercises, breathe out with your mouth open and imagine the muscles soft and relaxed. The more you can go with this feeling the easier it will be for you. Your conscious awareness and your breathing will be an invaluable support to birth your baby now. You are empowered and strong and your body is open, surrendering to the birth of your baby.

Feel you are like a flower opening to the sun.

The desire to push can be overwhelming. There is no stopping the natural urge to bear down and you will want to respond with an as yet unrealised force and extraordinary strength that comes from within you. You will breathe intuitively here and the more you can use the power within the breath and your mind, the more energy you will be giving to your body. The birth attendants will be guiding you when to push and where, and how to breathe most effectively. Remember there is a time to push and a time not to push. Using force at the wrong moment can delay the delivery and sometimes result in tearing. You might find it helpful to groan, moan, yell or hum as you bear down, using the sound to help the effort and lessen pain.

After each contraction rest where you have the opportunity and go to your baby with thoughts of love and encouragement. The moment when you meet for the first time is so near now. Clear your mind and prepare for the next powerful urge, each one bringing you closer. When it is time, breathe your baby into the world as gently as possible.

Third Stage

The third stage of labour is when the placenta is delivered. Most women want to leave the cord attached until it has stopped pulsing. Cutting the cord is the first of many natural separations that

171

occur between mother and baby, of letting go gently, little by little.

There is a lot of interest in what to do with the placenta. It depends on where you have your baby and your feelings about the placenta. Some women are happy to leave it at the hospital, others like to take it home and bury it under a tree in the garden. This is a gesture of giving back to the earth—as the earth has provided nourishment for you during pregnancy, in many ways it seems fitting to nourish the earth in return. In some cultures part of the placenta is eaten by the new mother as it is considered to be very high in the nutrients most needed after giving birth.

A practice which is becoming more popular is Lotus Birth, where the cord is left uncut and connected to the placenta. The placenta is washed and salted daily and placed in a container, or in a bag often made especially for the purpose, until the cord separates from it, which can happen as soon as three days after the birth or take as long as 10 days. The placenta is usually buried afterward. The belief here is that the energy from the placenta is still important to the baby and mother and that it is a more gentle approach than cutting the cord at birth (see Sarah Buckley, *Gentle Birth, Gentle Mothers*). In my experience with my sons' births I felt the cutting of the cord was a separation on the physical level only. It was the first of many such moments as they grew and became their own persons, but the spiritual connection we share, as mother and child, will never be severed on any level.

There have been rituals involving the placenta other than Lotus Birth since time began. This list comes from Catherine Price and Sandra Robinson's wonderful book, *Birth: Conceiving, Nurturing and Giving Birth to Your Baby*:

- Aborigines use the cord to make necklaces for the child to wear to ward off disease.
- The Sudanese consider the placenta to be the infant's 'spirit double' and it is buried in a place that represents the parents' hopes for their child, e.g. close to a hospital to become a doctor.
- In Yemen the placenta is placed on the family's roof for the birds to eat, in the hope that it will guarantee love between the parents.
- Malaysians see the placenta as the child's other sibling, with the two being reunited at death. The midwife carefully washes it and wraps it in a white cloth to be buried.
- The Chinese consider the placenta a powerful medicine. It is dried and powdered and placed in capsules for the woman to take at various times in her life, including menopause (page 303).

CHAPTER 20

AFFIRMATIONS, VISUALISATIONS AND MANAGING PAIN

Empowering Words and Affirmations

The use of affirmations in the form of a single word or a statement helps maintain the connection between you, your most positive and needed energies, and your baby. While there are many excellent books written on the benefit of affirmations, it is worth spending a little time composing your own, as they will have a more personal feel. Always choose words that are positive and thus promote the feelings you most want. Never use words such as 'fear', 'panic', 'anxiety' or 'pain' or phrases that focus on what you don't want, such as 'am not', 'have not', 'might be'. This is especially relevant if you have had a previous pregnancy and birthing experience that was difficult in some way. Concentrate on the present moment and work with the positive energy available to you now, rather than relive a past experience that was fearful and carry negative energy into this birth experience. Take some time to resolve any negative or frightening experience so that this time in your life can be fully embraced as new and positive. If the birth was traumatic, seek professional counselling to help you move on to the present with confidence and courage. In such a case affirmations are helpful in conjunction with counselling, but are not enough on their own.

The affirmations can be said out loud, repeated to yourself, or written down and read on waking, during the day and before sleep. Some people find it very helpful to write their affirmations a number of times each day until they are comfortable with the 'feel' of them, changing the words until they resonate better.

Birth is a natural process—I embrace the energy of birth.

I flow with the natural process of birth.

I am a beautiful woman, my body and mind express radiance and love.

I am calm and at peace with myself.

I love being a woman, I love my pregnant body.

I will birth (am birthing) my baby easily and gently.

I am open to the process of labour and birth.

I am calm and at peace with my new life as a mother.

I welcome and accept the changes in my body and the new life growing in my womb.

I am loved, and feel love in every part of my life.

I am safe, supported and loved.

I love and appreciate myself as I am.

I trust the natural process of birth.

I surrender to the energy of birth.

I accept and embrace the birthing process.

To the baby … I love you. You are welcome, you are loved. You are my precious baby.

Here are a few examples of affirmations for pregnancy and labour (see box). Spend some time thinking about what feels right for you, and use them as a guide to creating your own.

Or just use single powerful words that are relevant to you—for example, *open … peace … calm … soft … gentle … courage … power … strength.*

Sometimes the best power words and affirmations come to you intuitively during quiet inner reflection. Write them down and use them regularly in meditation as an important part of your birth preparation. The more you think about them and practise them while you are pregnant, the easier it will be to bring them to mind during labour. Encourage your partner and other birth support people to become familiar with your power words and affirmations so they can remind you of them during labour, especially if you become vague or disorientated.

Father's Affirmations

Sometimes the father of the baby feels a bit detached or disconnected from the whole pregnancy, for the simple reasons that he is not carrying the baby and his view of things is quite different from the mother's. But the father's role is of course very important, and it is appropriate that he creates some affirmations of his own—a few simple words of special relevance to him, perhaps in reference to his role as a father and a parent or his deep inner feelings towards his baby. This will give him another way to communicate and bond with his baby before the birth, just as the mother is doing.

The flower meditation is a powerful image to keep in your mind during labour because of what it symbolises and because it really encourages women to open to birth their baby. Some women have a real flower with them during labour, others have an artificial one, some even have a photo.

The meditation on Your Baby's Light, visualising your baby being filled with light or with light around her, or maybe light in the birth canal, has also used successfully during the birthing process. Using colour in meditation appeals to many women and during labour it helps to maintain balance and harmony, and to feel safe and protected. Detailed visualisations are outlined in chapter 14, Creative meditations and visualisation.

Many women respond favourably visualising a special place in nature, or a place that has particular relevance for them. The mere thought makes them feel calm and safe, and this can be a very useful technique to remember during labour. When a woman chooses a beautiful and peaceful place from her own experiences or from her imagination, she can relate to it personally and become more completely involved.

My client Lindsay used this technique to great benefit during her labour. Whenever we did this meditation in class, she would imagine herself in the nature reserve behind her home, which is a beautiful and serene place. In pre-labour she went for a walk in the reserve with her husband and this helped her to stay calm and relaxed. Later on, in the final stages, she again focused on this special place and found it helped her stay composed and in the moment. It is a true example of bringing the world of imagery into the real world. Other women take a photo of their special place with them into the delivery suite. In a similar way the Tree meditation, or imagining the calmness of water, can be used to give you strength and courage and to help you feel grounded and connected with the physical energies required for birth.

Positions for Labour

The positions you use during labour will depend entirely on your unique circumstances and on what you find the most comfortable. If your labour is straightforward you will be free to be active and change position when ever you choose. When circumstances prevent you making a change to your position, you will need to follow the guidance of your health professionals.

What you do is very much a personal choice, especially as the positions you find yourself in often occur quite spontaneously. You might also find yourself in a posture you least expected to be beneficial. Not all women want to move during labour, even if labour is progressing well.

There are a few positions that are used consistently and are worth trying, even if not for the duration. If you find one position is good for a while but then is no longer working for you, always move to another one.

Gravity plays an important part in labour. Helpful upright positions include leaning against the wall or against your birth support, standing and leaning over a bed or even the kitchen bench if you are still at home. Pelvic rocking while standing is recommended for both pain relief and the benefits of gravity. Squatting is ideal if you find it comfortable as you are in the best birth position anatomically, with gravity working perfectly. However, you need to be familiar with squatting and reasonably strong in your legs to maintain it for any length of time. If squatting is comfortable but too tiring, a semi-squatting position utilising a stool, a low step or even a pile of books is far less exhausting but still provides all the benefits. Or try holding onto a table or bench and squat down from that position. Birthing chairs and exercise balls, used for comfort and the benefits of gravity, are available at most hospitals.

A supported squatting position is excellent and can be done with the birth support seated facing you, supporting you under the arms or holding your hands, while you are either in a full squatting position or on a low stool; or your birth support is seated, while you squat facing away. If you are both standing, your birth support holds you under the arms. This last suggestion is a good option but can be very hard on the one holding you, especially if the position needs to be maintained for a long time. If you have two birth supports, stand with one person on each side holding you under the arms.

Resting on your hands and knees is excellent if you have backache, and especially if the baby is in an occipito-posterior position, where her back and skull are resting against your sacrum. This can be extremely uncomfortable. Spending time on hands and knees often brings welcome relief as it draws the weight of the baby away from your spine, almost as if the pressure has vanished, relaxing the whole pelvic area.

Women enjoy pelvic rocking on all fours during labour, making big slow circles either during a contraction or in preparation for the next one. These slow relaxed movements release tension throughout the hips, lower back and pelvis. The breathing can be synchronised, one breath coordinated with one slow circle. This is very relaxing and centring having a mesmerising effect as you rock slowly and breathe in rhythm. When the contraction has finished you can rest in the Child Pose to prepare for the next one. Moving during labour has a positive effect on reducing pain and prevents the muscles from becoming too tense and rigid.

Bean bags mould to your body shape and are a good choice for labour. You can lean on the bean bag from the hands and knees position or have it behind you so that can sit back to rest after the contraction. Two of them can mean double the comfort. Leaning over a bed on your knees is also very comfortable. Leaning positions make it easier for your birth support to massage your back.

A supported semi-inclined seated position is often preferred for labour and delivery, with the knees drawn close up to the chest in a 'frog' position and your feet resting on the birth support, sometimes with one on each side of you. From this position your legs are able to fall freely out to the sides and relax, especially if they feel shaky and weak as labour advances. Massage of your inner thighs in this position gives wonderful relief and draws your awareness down the body. You can sit in a bean bag, on a bed, or on the floor with cushions for comfort, or with your birth support sitting behind you. The semi-inclined position is sometimes used during a water birth, as is the all fours position. From this position a mirror can be held which will allow you to see your body opening to birth your baby.

Lying on your side with cushions under your head and your abdomen, and between your legs, is also suitable and very functional for labour and delivery.

Managing Pain

Everybody has a different pain threshold. You may have encountered pain on several previous occasions, but the feelings experienced during labour are very different. While some women liken it to strong period pain, every labour is different. I am hesitant to use the word 'pain' when talking about labour and childbirth, as it can immediately create tension and recall unpleasant images or memories. Some women prefer to call contractions 'surges of the uterine muscles', or 'waves'; if one of these terms feels better for you, remember to use it during the birthing process. But whatever you call the intense physical feelings of labour, the management of those feelings is what is important.

Your attitude toward pain, and what you consider your pain threshold to be, will have a significant influence on how you deal with the pain of childbirth. If you are positive and relaxed about giving birth, and

The Role of Hormones

Your body truly is wondrous. Unless there is a physical reason or complications that will prevent you from birthing a baby, as a woman you are made to do so. If you are in the situation where your body initiates labour naturally, it will release the perfect sequence of hormones to support you through labour and birth. In brief these are:

Oxytocin is often called the hormone of love. Released during labour, it is involved in uterine contractions and heightened at birth helping you to open to birth and after birth to release the placenta. After the birth the oxytocin level is at its highest. Women often comment that it was love at first sight when they saw their baby. This is because they are flooded with the love hormone so that the bond between mother and baby is set in place at birth. Oxytocin is the hormone released during sex and orgasm, breast-feeding and whenever we have affectionate, warm sensations towards another. It is involved in the all aspects of the reproductive system. Synthetic oxytocin is used when labour is induced but because it is not naturally produced by the woman's body the responses are not the same during the birthing process. However, natural oxytocin is released as soon as a woman holds her baby and has skin to skin contact, and while breast-feeding.

Prostaglandin is released close to the time of birth and helps soften the cervix.

Prolactin, also referred to as the 'mothering hormone', is released at birth, which is important for the mother–baby bond to be set in place, and while breast-feeding.

Beta-endorphins are released as a natural form of pain relief, and are also present during breast-feeding.

Adrenaline and noradrenaline We all need adrenaline and noradrenaline, which are the hormones that come into play when we are frightened or in danger. They are known as the 'fight or flight' hormones. Adrenaline has an important role in the second stage of labour, helping the woman to be more alert as she prepares to give birth. If it is produced before this time it blocks the pain-reducing hormones—this can be caused by stress, or even loud noise, excess lighting and too much activity. This is why it is so important for a woman to be as relaxed as possible during labour and wherever possible to be in a calm and quiet environment.

willing to trust in yourself and your birth support, surrender totally to it and accept what the day brings, you are more likely to deal with what the time brings with an open mind and in an easier manner. You will experience labour and childbirth in a very different way than someone who is afraid, to whom the mere thought of pain brings anxiety and tension.

Having some fear around the birth is natural and quite realistic, because it is the great unknown, it is often painful and things can go wrong. There is also no judgement about choosing pain relief and for some women the only option at the time. Be aware that if you do use pain relief it is very easy to allow yourself to feel intimidated by others who didn't use it, or to have feelings of guilt and regret after the birth which are not going to benefit anyone, most especially you and your baby. You are you, and the birth of your baby is your experience, and yours alone.

Also be aware that there are too many people who are more than willing to tell you the most horrendous birth stories while you are pregnant—which does nothing to help you to feel positive and confident. Often these misplaced comments come from complete strangers who for whatever reason feel you need

to warned and need you to know their view on birthing. And yes, even though giving birth can be complicated and stressful, you are *not them* and this is *your experience.*

Be selective in what you listen to and don't be tempted to read too much about what can go wrong. There is a middle path to all things including childbirth. Be well informed and surround yourself with those who will support you and give good practical, honest advice. Listen to the birth stories that didn't go to plan but were still beautiful and positive, as well as to women who had a fulfilling experience, natural or otherwise, so you are encouraged and more optimistic.

The more centred and relaxed you are and the more mindful you are of your emotions and thoughts, the better you will manage what your labour brings. Remember to trust, surrender and accept so you go with the process of birthing more easily and more confidently.

It is natural to withdraw from pain and discomfort and to tighten and tense the corresponding muscles and be 'closed' in the cervix. Pain makes us tighten the shoulders and hands, clench the teeth, tighten the jaw, to breathe erratically or too shallow in the chest, and often to hold the breath. But during labour the

opposite is required. Going with the physical sensations you are feeling and breathing into and through the pain—in contrast to becoming tense and trying to distance yourself from it—the easier labour will be. If you can do this you will feel less discomfort because your body is relaxed and your mind is there with the sensations, and with your baby. When your attention is held firmly in the present moment and you are absorbed by what is happening in your body and how you are breathing, the more you will merge with the whole experience and then actively participate in the birth.

Some women feel it very helpful to 'colour' the intense feelings. Concentrate on the feelings, and then surround them with a healing colour so as to soften and disperse them with your imagination. Spend some time before your due date thinking about what might be the most useful and helpful for you, so when the time comes you are prepared and ready.

Movement can be an effective way of managing pain as it prevents the muscles from becoming tense and sore, and walking or pelvic rocking are possible options to keep the body relaxed through movement. A few acupressure points that are very effective for pain relief are discussed in the next chapter.

BIRTH STORIES

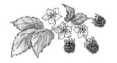

For me, pregnancy was an initiatory experience that changed my body, shifted my consciousness, taught me surrender, and was the beginning of the dawning awareness of the physical, psychological, and spiritual demands and gifts that would come through being a mother.

Jean Shinoda Bolen, *Crossing to Avalon*, page 53

It is my great pleasure to include these very personal stories from women who have practiced yoga during their pregnancies. As you will see, some women were very involved in yoga for the entire pregnancy, others discovered it only during the last few months, yet all felt it played an important role in childbirth. I hope they will prove to be valuable and insightful reading while you prepare for the birth of your baby.

When you are pregnant, it is very helpful to listen to other women speak about their birth experiences, especially how they handled the different stages of labour. It can help to build confidence and courage for your own special journey and relieve much of the mystery around childbirth.

Obviously, some labour stories are not as easy to listen to as others. Even if a birth is not straightforward and requires intervention it can still be a positive experience. For many women, giving birth is one of the most remarkable and inspiring times in their lives. For this reason, I encourage you to listen to all stories, even the inevitable 'horror' stories, and especially to seek out women who had a more positive and fulfilling time, and to draw strength from their encouraging experience. Finding the balance between all the possibilities of pregnancy, labour and childbirth, and being in touch with the realities of life, will prepare you for your experience.

My Story

The idea for this book came about when I was pregnant with my first son Ezra. I had been practising yoga for many years and continuing on with it during pregnancy seemed the logical thing to do. At that time I was fortunate enough to be under the guidance of an excellent teacher, Swami Shantimurti, and I spoke to him about a specific yoga program that would prepare my body for conception, the changes that would occur during pregnancy and as a birth preparation. I wanted to be as healthy and strong as I could be before conception, not only through a healthy diet and lifestyle but also with the assistance of yoga.

To complete my naturopathic studies at a college in Auckland I was required to do a thesis. I remember knowing I wanted to do mine on yoga and pregnancy and I was thrilled when Angela, the lecturer in charge of thesis topics, accepted my choice.

And so began my long journey with this book. To complete more studies in Australia I provided an enlarged and more detailed update of the original thesis, which became the background for this book. In many ways the book has had its own growth in utero as it slowly took

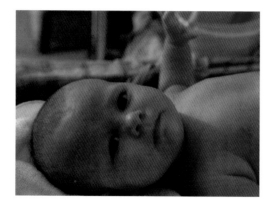

form over time, growing and developing, maturing and becoming whole, until its 'birth' when it was finally completed.

My own experience with yoga began in Melbourne where I attended classes for some years. Later on, I had the opportunity to delve deeper while travelling in India particularly in the extraordinary city of Bombay, now known by the original name Mumbai, and then later while living in London. After returning to Australia for a brief time, I moved to New Zealand and unexpectedly found myself teaching a large group in a provincial town, which continued for a couple of years before moving to Auckland where I met one of my most influential teachers, Shantimurti and later Bhaktimurti.

My initiation into teaching yoga for pregnancy seemed to come about as something I was meant to do rather than something I had the time to actually consider. After a happy and healthy pregnancy and a fairly straightforward birth with Ezra using my yoga breathing practices and postures, my doctor

suggested—while I was still in the delivery room—that I start classes for pregnant women as soon as I was ready. It was not really something I was thinking about 15 minutes after giving birth however, his suggestion that day became a small class of women six months later who were all referred by him. That was in 1984.

My second son, Reuben, was to have quite a different experience from his brother both in utero and for his birth. We were living aboard our yacht when I conceived and we were sailing the Pacific during the last five months of his pregnancy. Due to engine problems we were forced to stop for repairs at the island of Espiritu Santo in northern Vanuatu when I was about 32 weeks.

On visiting the very basic and unsophisticated local hospital there, I was told by the local doctor that he would not interfere with the birth as this was the domain of the midwives and that there were no analgesics handed out for normal deliveries. He told me that in Vanuatu, if a caesarean was required the incision was from the top of the abdomen to the pubic bone. He also told me no real fuss was made about labour and birth in Vanuatu because women had babies all the time and they just got on with it as well as they could. Although I realise that giving birth and having babies is a very natural part of life and something that does happen all the time, it was still a bit of a shock that his approach was so simplistic. So being forewarned with the reality of the

situation, I armed myself with all the skills I knew, practising my yoga postures and especially the breathing exercises and daily meditation intensely for the remaining 8 weeks of my pregnancy.

I also knew that it was considered taboo for men to be present at the birth in Vanuatu and without that support from my husband Jeff, I had to find all the strength I needed from within myself. With this to consider I relied heavily on meditation and visualisation techniques, the yoga postures I had enjoyed the most as well as plain positive thinking, all of which I feel played a big part in what turned out to be a very straightforward delivery. I used the deep yoga breathing leading into a contraction and after it has eased away, and sometimes deep cleansing breaths to blow away tension and to clear my mind. I also relied on having my breath and firm awareness in the abdomen, breathing out through my mouth which kept me focused, relaxed and my attention with Reuben. My favourite breathing had always been the ujjayi technique in its traditional form as well as with deep breathing etc. and found it held me in a clear and present mind space and was an excellent focus point. I also relied on simple breath awareness, being as conscious as possible of the natural breath and importantly the potential in it. These breathing practices were what helped me stay centred and calm and even though I had been practicing yoga and teaching it for some time, it was very apparent to me just how valuable these simple practices were and how they were really working for me, they were even more important and beneficial than I had realised. Maybe I was lucky, but I know I would not have handled such unusual circumstances or been so relaxed, if I had not physically, and most importantly, mentally and emotionally, prepared myself beforehand with yoga and trusted in these techniques as my labour progressed.

I have warm and pleasant memories of the day Reuben was born. I was feeling very relaxed about what was happening and felt so calm as I progressed through the contractions, completely focused on my breathing and going with the whole birthing process. I was definitely helped out by nature on that cool September evening. For most of the first stage I was on the beach where the yacht was moored then, later that evening, I moved through the more intense contractions on the hill outside the hospital which overlooked the sea, a lot of the time leaning against a coconut tree for support and gravity to assist me. All the while, I was being cooled by a light breeze that swayed the coconut palms. In many ways it was perfect, just me and Reuben moving through the birthing process together in this quiet natural setting.

My circumstances meant that this labour was going to be very different from Ezra's but it was a very calm and peaceful experience. I was able to become absorbed in the natural birthing processes and connect with my inner feminine wisdom and be there completely with Reuben. I believe this situation gave me the courage to trust in my body and to surrender to the way my labour was progressing, and was how I truly came to realise the incredible potential of yoga.

I am especially grateful for the knowledge that yoga played such a significant role in helping me manage and for Reuben to come into the world in a calm and gentle way.

There were definitely no luxuries offered at that small hospital, not even a cup of tea, a warm shower after the delivery or a bath for Reuben so we came back to the boat early the next day for a peaceful time together with our new family member, on the still waters of Pelacula Bay. Although we had no family or friends there to visit us and welcome Reuben to the world, we did receive radio calls from other boats in the Pacific area, wishing us all well and Reuben welcome aboard. Reuben lived the first 12 months of his life on the water before we moved back onto land and it was not long after that I began teaching again.

I have been teaching yoga and meditation to pregnant women since 1984 and hope to continue this work for many years to come. Yoga has always been a strong and supportive base for women during their pregnancies and as a birth preparation and over the years has grown and developed into a simple and very useable structure. I have complete faith and trust in the practices, especially as I have seen how incredibly valuable they have been to so many women including myself. I often wonder at how fortunate I am to be in the remarkable position of teaching yoga as a profession and especially to have the good fortune to be teaching women at such a unique and precious time in their lives. Not only do I love this work and see it more as a blessing than a job, but it has also given me the opportunity to meet and make close friends with many beautiful and inspiring women, who have taught me so much more about the value of yoga during the brief time of their pregnancies. Of course, there is the additional joy of finally meeting their newborns, often only days after being born and occasionally being at the birth of a new life. It is always a very emotional experience for me after observing them move and grow in their mother's abdomen for so many months.

Natalie's Three Boys

When I fell pregnant with my first child I felt that I needed to prepare myself not only for the birth but for the pregnancy itself. I simply couldn't just turn up on the day and thrust that all would go well. Therefore I took the opportunity to try a yoga class. It quickly changed the way I thought and felt about my body and gave me an incredible connection to my growing baby. I so enjoyed my first experience that I continued to practice

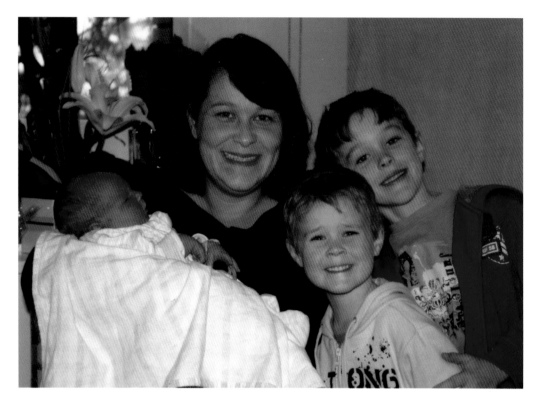

Genevieve's Story

I started yoga with Theresa when I was about 20 weeks pregnant with my third child. I was unable to exercise earlier due to a few problems so yoga seemed the logical choice. I needed a calm and relaxing approach to birth and I found the classes such a calming experience in comparison to my hectic life with two small children while they also allowed some time with my growing baby. Another great aspect of these classes was the interaction with other pregnant woman who were sharing their pregnancy journeys with me. I especially liked the pelvic rocking on all fours and the Child Pose as these were very comfortable and relieved a lot of pressure from my back. I told Theresa I was going to spend some of my labour in the Sleeping Tortoise due to the wonderful relief it gave my back and thighs, and I did just that right up until the time came for me to push. I went in to labour two weeks early, I had strong contractions at home then my waters broke and I went straight to hospital. Once in hospital I headed to the shower and began deep squats and standing pelvic rocking to relieve back pain and to keep my body and baby moving. All the time I visualised a lily opening as an image of my cervix dilating as we had done in class. I did these movements and the visualisation to try and progress quickly and further into my labour. I moved to the spa and sat with my belly sitting in the warm water in the child pose as this gave me

yoga for my three pregnancies and in between too. As well as the practices I also shared this experience with many other wonderful new mums and made great friends along the way. I learnt how to breathe, stretch, relax and focus my attention where I needed it most. I also used many of the yoga positions to relieve discomfort during pregnancy and during labour. I was able to focus on my breathing and completely relax between contractions and I could visualise opening my pelvis and helping my baby to be born. Through using the yoga practices during these times I gained an enormous strength within myself that I never realised I had before. I felt empowered and am proud that I have dealt with the intensity of labour and given birth to my three sons

naturally. After each birth I continued to use the throat breath and humming to relax and calm my babies who I'm sure responded to the familiar sounds. Both my older sons would hum themselves to sleep. I also discovered how to relax and let go of tension in my body to allow my milk to flow easily while breast feeding. I have learnt so many valuable lessons that I continue to practice everyday. I believe that Theresa has created such a wonderful environment through her classes for so many of us expectant mothers. Practicing yoga during my pregnancies has enriched this very special time in my life and I will remember the beautiful times that I shared with each of my babies before they were born and after as well.

wonderful relief from back discomfort and also gave the rest of my body some rest. I had intended having a water birth but after only a short time in the spa I became very hot and flushed so I went back to the shower and continued with more pelvic rocking while standing and on my hands and knees. During this time I also leant against the wall of the shower to stretch my calf muscles and relieve my back. The contractions became quite intense so I gathered my thoughts and energy and sat in the sleeping tortoise again and continued with the lily visualisation and my cervix opening to birth my baby. When the contractions became too painful I rolled over onto my hands and knees, with my head in a pillow clenching my husbands hands. I breathed slowly and

deeply and within 10 minutes I could feel my baby coming. I gave a few pushes and my beautiful baby girl Isabelle was born. The labour was a total of 2 hours 50 minutes and drug free. I had achieved the calm and controlled birth experience I had hoped for and felt elated with my baby daughter. Even though my labour was relatively fast it was also very intense and I was so pleased with how well I had handled my self. As well as this I now have a wonderful group of friends from my yoga classes who I catch up every fortnight, which is great for us and our babies have friends of their own age too. We have been a great support to each other and are sure we will be friends for the rest of our lives.

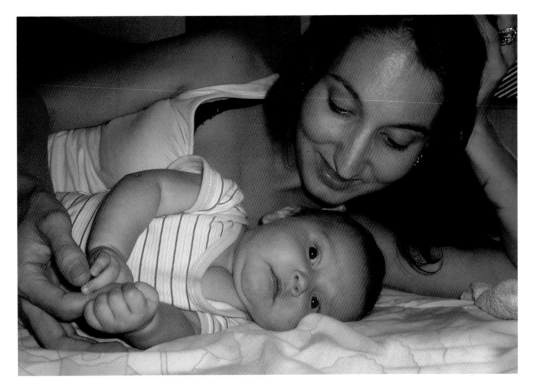

Storm Boy

My husband and I were very excited as we prepared for the birth of our first child. As the weeks passed we were made aware that our baby was in the frank breech position. Our Obstetrician was very clear in explaining that a vaginal delivery was not an option. Should our baby not turn to a head down position a caesarian section would be scheduled. I have always expected that I would have a vaginal delivery – a caesarian section never entered my mind as an option for me..

At 37.5 weeks gestation I was lying wide awake struggling to fall asleep and listening to the rain pound on our tin roof. It was the sort of tropical rain common to the Queensland Hinterland. At this time I felt an unusual release of fluid. Both my husband and I soon realised that our baby was deciding his time was right to greet the world. We called the hospital and were advised to venture down the Mountain to have the situation assessed. The rain continued to pound the roof.

We commenced a slow drive down the Mountain with visibility limited and much debris across our path. I reminded myself to focus on my own breathing as we crossed a flooded section of road with the water gushing at the headlights of the car. We then came to another section of flooded road, this time it was evident that the flow was rapid, the current strong. I calmly yet forcefully said "We can not cross this". Subsequently several forms of rescue vehicles – car, truck and boat also

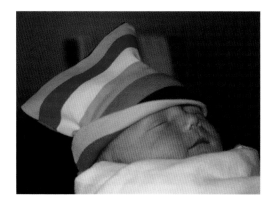

felt that indeed this gushing waterway was bigger than them.

It now became obvious that the first flooded section of road was impassable. We were trapped between two flooded creeks! It was 1.00am. Both our mobile phones had no signal. Unable to go forward or turn back we selected a nearby house in order to use a landline phone and seek shelter.

We were out of the elements and we were safe. My aim was clear, I had to keep myself calm and focus on the fact that I was in a warm and protected environment. I knew I had to do this in order to keep my baby safe.

For the next 3.5 hours a stranger's spare room was my place of refuge. I lay still on the bed in the dark and remained calm and at peace . I knew I had the tools to do this as I had been practising them in weekly meditation classes for the previous six weeks. I used these tools to calmly and consciously create an inner stillness as the storm continued to rage outside. I had my breath to focus on. I used "throat breathing" and "counting the breath" as

the main techniques. During this period my husband was in constant contact with emergency services and various medical staff, he could sense that I was surprisingly still and calm.

The hours passed surprisingly quickly, it seemed as if it had been mere minutes rather than hours when a four-wheel drive ambulance finally came to our rescue. I was extremely relieved. I had been feeling more tightening sensations in my lower abdomen and was so very pleased to be heading to the hospital. The paramedic took my vitals and was impressed to find that my blood pressure was in the normal range. It remained this way as we made our way to the hospital along a bumpy road down the mountain. We stopped at times as the competent crew advised other motorists of the dangers ahead and to clear the road of fallen tree branches.

The journey came to an end 1.5 hours later and I have never been so happy to see a hospital. We were all safe. I was assessed and ready for the birth of our baby. I was dilated and my baby was in no distress, the caesarian section was performed 30 minutes later. He chose his time to enter the world and we his parents had the joy and celebration of his arrival. I have no doubt that the meditative state I was able to go into provided this positive outcome.

Therese's Girls:
Allana and Makeisha

I started doing yoga in my first pregnancy when I was working a high pressure job

and found it very fulfilling attending every week. It was my time for me. I also made time to go to classes in my second pregnancy and found it was my time to nurture myself and this amazing gift growing inside of me. While attending these classes I met a group of women who are now very good friends and are a support to each other and I would not have this great network if I had not attended yoga.

The births of my two children were entirely different and I want to share my stories as I found that listening to other women's experiences and reading about them helped me keep an open mind as to what might happened during labour and birth. Allana was five weeks early which was a big shock, I never imagined having a premature baby especially as we had just moved house that day and my waters broke early that evening. I had mild contractions for about four hours before I realised we had better go to hospital. I did some yoga postures from the classes and found the humming quite calming as it gave me something to focus on. I did pelvic rocking which was most beneficial to relieve backache and rested in the child pose in between contractions. I also spent time in the spa to relieve pain in my back and my legs and did a lot of humming during that time also. I had wanted a drug free birth but just 'hit the wall' and asked for some pain relief. I used gas and a lot of humming to help me through transition and then around 4 am our darling baby

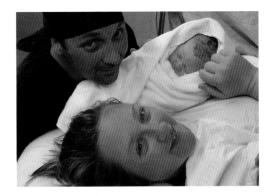

daughter was born a healthy 6 pounds 4 ounces.

The arrival of Makeisha was completely different. She attempted to be born nine weeks early but as my waters hadn't broken the doctor was able to slow things down. I was ordered to rest until at least 37 weeks and surprisingly I managed to follow these orders. I was concerned she was going to be a big baby because Allana was a good size even though she was five weeks early, and used acupuncture and other natural therapies to hopefully

give birth any time after 37 weeks. But Makeisha had other plans and wasn't ready until I was a week overdue. I was induced and was hoping for a quick delivery and to have a water birth. I got into the birthing pool and did a lot of pelvic rocking because she was posterior and I was having a lot of back pain. I found humming helped again as it did the first time and after seven hours in the pool I asked for my waters to be broken. It then became very intense and the doctor tried using the vacuum to help her be born, but this was not effective. In fact I was having what is known as an 'obstructive labour' and I was told she needed to be born by caesarean. I did my best to remain calm especially when the epidural was given and found it very helpful to use some other breathing exercises including ujjayi breathing. She was born a very healthy 9 pounds 11 ounces. I found yoga to

be very nurturing and valuable for both pregnancies and births and I will certainly be doing it again for any children we have in the future.

Debbie's Story: The Birth of Callan

As this was my first child, I wanted to prepare myself and I felt yoga would be the most ideal way to cater to the mental and physical demands of pregnancy and childbirth. I joined Theresa's yoga group at about 18 weeks into my pregnancy. The classes were designed for pregnancy, so the postures, meditation and relaxation techniques were ideally suited and specific to the needs of an advancing pregnancy. Also, you were able to work at your own level and pace which I feel is important.

The benefits were almost immediate, particularly if you were disciplined and practised at home on a daily basis. The interaction with other pregnant ladies was great and also quite social. My intention was to continue the classes until I was due, but Mother Nature was to chart her own course as I developed pregnancy-induced hypertension at 26 weeks.

At 32 weeks I was hospitalised, and the challenge I was faced with was to try and extend my pregnancy for as long as possible. It was at this point that yoga became particularly important for me, as I was surrounded by women having their babies and then going home. Quite the opposite for me, however, as I was trying very hard not to have my baby and at the same time pass my time in hospital

---

Author's note: The midwife told Therese after the birth that although she had gone through all stages of labour her baby was pushing forcefully on the walls of the cervix for many hours thereby causing swelling and obstructing the opening of the cervix, making a natural birth impossible as this had progressed too far. This is known as an obstructed labour and in Therese's situation a caesarean was a necessity and life saving. Obstructed labour is unfortunately very common in many underprivileged countries and with devastating consequences. If you are interested in knowing more about this, I recommend Catherine Hamlin's book, *The Hospital by the River: A Story of Hope*. This inspiring true story is about the wonderful work done by a husband and wife doctor team who have dedicated their lives to reducing this problem for poor village women in Africa.

effectively and positively. So yoga became a very big part of my daily routine in hospital, and as it turned out enabled me to remain calm mentally, which in turn kept my blood pressure levels sufficiently low to gain valuable weeks for my baby to continue to grow and develop, until I was induced at 36 weeks.

During the initial stages of labour, I walked a lot and then retired to the spa in the birthing suite and seriously concentrated on the breathing techniques I had learnt at the yoga classes. I choose to spend a lot of this time alone, which allowed my mind to be incredibly focused and clear and afforded me a degree of control physically, to work with the contractions as my labour progressed to the transitional stage. At this point, I left

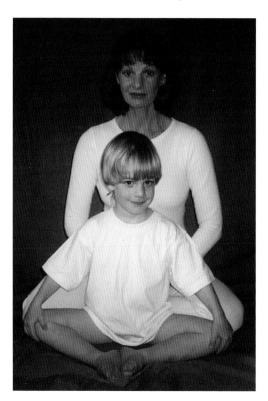

the spa and tried various positions on the floor, maintaining my breathing the whole time. From transition to the actual birth, everything proceeded very quickly and my husband and girlfriend joined me to witness the wondrous moment our baby boy arrived, healthy and beautiful. My labour was drug free which amazed me, as I am certainly no martyr and had decided, in advance, to take pain relief if and when I needed it.

A few days after the birth my midwife asked me if I would speak to her current ante natal class before I went home. I inquired why, and she told me that I had gone into a trance like state as soon as I got into the spa, concentrating on deep breathing, and remaining that way the entire time. She felt it was my knowledge of yoga that rewarded me with a very easy labour, as labour goes, and wanted me to share this with her class, which I did happily. Upon reflection, I now realise what an 'out of body experience' my labour had been, even though I was not aware of this at the time.

To be honest I thought my yoga had served its purpose during pregnancy and labour, so I moved on to the busy days ahead caring for our son, Callan. No one can really prepare you for labour, you must experience it. The same applies to the first weeks at home, when the days roll into nights of very little sleep and you seem to merely exist for your baby, constantly wondering if what you are doing is correct, while at the same time

becoming familiar with your baby. It is during these early weeks you are really tested mentally and physically. Once again yoga came to my rescue and I was able to draw on my ability through meditation to remain calm mentally, and the relaxation techniques boosted me physically and emotionally.

Overall, I am convinced yoga was my saviour at times when I needed it most and still is on a daily basis, proving to me the benefits of yoga don't cease with labour. Applied daily or as often as time allows, yoga in all its forms continues to feed the mind, body and soul, at a time when our lives become so busy and stressful. In turn this flows on to contribute to a contented baby, so mother and father can both be more relaxed to enjoy the new role of parenting. I feel everyone should have access to the benefits of yoga if they so desire, especially during pregnancy.

Trish: The Birth of Ebony-Jayne

My son was born 10 years earlier in a relatively short time, lasting only four hours from the first twinge of labour to less than an hour for the second stage, and all my friends teased me saying I needed to experience a 'real birth'. Even though at that time, I was extremely fit and had been active up until the birth, I found that I needed to use gas as I had not learned to calm and control myself during the pregnancy. When it came to the final minutes of the birth, my mind wandered and focused on the pain, hence the tensing of muscles and the need to be cut to allow the baby free. Even though all births are a wonderful experience, taking the time to learn to relax the mind and body throughout this pregnancy, made the comparison between both births obvious.

The birth of our daughter Ebony-Jayne was a wonderful experience, even though my labour lasted a total of 17 hours, definitely a 'real birth', after being induced due to the rise in my blood pressure. I went into true labour quite excited after a false labour lasting 10 days, when I had lost the mucus plug and had been mildly labouring ever since with several false starts. I was now pleased my contractions were coming at a regular 7 to 10 minutes apart. My labour was progressing slowly and my friend Sharon gave me homeopathic drops, which helped the intensity of the contractions. After trying several positions for labour, I found lying on my side the most comfortable. After much time and really getting nowhere fast, my waters were broken by my doctor and from then on the contractions were close together and very intense, as well as the desire to push. I found that the pain was easier to handle on my hands and knees, relaxing into the Child Pose in between contractions to allow the weight and gravity to take the pressure off my back.

At this point there was a change of shifts and Tina became my midwife, a calm and skilled woman who encouraged me to breathe through the pain of each contraction. I wanted to push, but Tina told me I had at least 10 contractions to go, at which point my strength waned and I felt I couldn't last the distance—really telling myself I can't do this! But I pulled myself together and concentrated on the breathing I had been taught in yoga class, relaxing while breathing in and releasing all pain and discomfort while breathing out. I was able to push the panic I was feeling away, and started to relax as much as possible. Tina was encouraging me all the way, telling me to continue with what I was doing, but if I was to push at that time the baby's head would push against the cervix causing it to swell, which could cause complications if the swelling became too great. I remember Theresa telling me that the Mountain pose in a modified version was an effective way to relieve that pressure, as it allowed the baby to move slightly away from the cervix, reducing extra pressure and also my desire to push. So at the start of the next contraction in the all fours position, I straightened my legs and breathed and breathed and breathed. The overwhelming desire to push lessened as the baby fell with gravity away from the cervix, and after two more contractions Tina said I could push as I was completely dilated.

So I began to push and after several contractions my husband Brett said, 'I can see the head.' With Sharon on one side whispering encouragement and Dianne on the other massaging my back to relieve the pain—a pain I can only relate to a Chinese

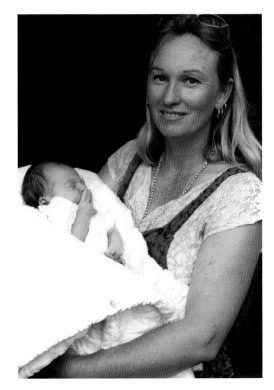

burn—Ebony came into the world with no tears, no stitches or drugs. A healthy 7 pound 2 ounce baby girl. They handed my beautiful daughter to me and as I focused on her I felt an enormous resurgence of energy, and I cried tears of love, joy, exhaustion and relief as I realised I had a daughter, Ebony-Jayne.

I then put her to my breast to encourage the birth of the placenta. Ebony's cord had now stopped pulsating and Brett cut the umbilical cord while she was in my arms, the joy and trepidation on his face was obvious as he hesitated, fearing he would hurt this tiny perfect baby who had just been born to us. He then held her in his arms and bonded with her. Tina pressed down onto the abdomen and the placenta was delivered in a few minutes, being a wonderful experience both physically and emotionally, a completion and cleansing after the whole birthing process. I recommend all women be allowed to enjoy this part of birth as naturally as possible, without the use of hormones to hurry on the process. Ebony's placenta is now feeding a candlenut tree that continues to grow in our yard, Ebony's tree.

I recommend yoga to any pregnant woman, for the benefits it gives to the body and the mind.

> **Author's note:** Tina Neff was the midwife attending Trish, for the birth of Ebony and she wrote this report about the experience.

I had the privilege of assisting Trish and Brett in the birth of their beautiful daughter, Ebony-Jayne. Once Trish was established in labour, she worked extremely well with her support person Dianne. During this time, she was encouraged to remain focused on her breathing and spontaneously changed positions to be on all fours. Even though Trish's labour was intense, she was able to remain in control and focus on her deeper rhythmic breathing. This control and focus certainly did a great deal to aid the process of labour.

Trish did so well with her breathing and focusing, that I would encourage anyone and everyone who is contemplating yoga training during their pregnancies, to certainly follow it through. Both the inner control and positioning greatly assisted Trish and Brett in achieving a wonderful birth experience.

Trish's support person, Dianne, also did a lot of back massage which helped in relaxing the back muscles and shifted the focus off the 'pain'. Stimulating the sacral points also helped to dissipate the pain and shift the centre of focus. A pain that is more 'dilute' and not so concentrated, is easier to deal with and get through.

After being privileged enough to assist Trish and Brett in their labour experience and share the wonderful, joyous moments of Ebony's birth, I would thoroughly and wholeheartedly recommend the practice of yoga and the breathing techniques to everyone. I can see that it not only assists in managing labour and birth, but also aides the person's inner strength and wellbeing.

Wendy Allen:
Sarah Joy Allen's 'Birth Day'

Sarah's conception was a honeymoon surprise. Delighted as I was, I knew nothing of what to expect of pregnancy or babies. So this was the beginning of an enormous and continuing learning experience. I wanted to have as healthy and natural pregnancy and birth as possible, and I focused on my physical and spiritual wellbeing. Yoga and hypnotherapy played a major part in my preparation program along with a healthy life style, with particular attention to diet and exercise.

Sarah's expected date of arrival, 20th of August, came and went. Rob and I saw our doctor after every five day's, and after two and a half weeks of waiting we decided to induce Sarah on the 6th of September. Over those final days of waiting we exhausted all the natural methods of inducement including hypnotherapy, yoga, acupuncture, massage, lots of exercise, lovemaking and wishful thinking!

On the evening of the 5th, after checking into the hospital, the nurses inserted the progesterone jelly at 10 p.m. and 4 a.m. My contractions were slow and I found I was able to use various yoga poses during this time, including Squatting and the Butterfly Pose in particular. At 1 p.m. my doctor arrived and as things were progressing very slowly, my waters were broken and the drip was inserted. I thought I was prepared for this but I found myself feeling very uncomfortable, anxious and fearful. Once the drip was inserted the show started without me, and the intensity of the pain took me by surprise.

At this time I really wanted a caesarean, but the strength and compassion I found in Joy's voice [the midwife] convinced me I didn't need one or really want one. She gave me the faith and strength I needed in myself and everything changed from that moment on. I realised I had to help myself and that I was going nowhere with my negativity, accepting there was no way out but forward, being strong and positive.

All the techniques I had learnt in the previous months came flooding back to me, and I became focused on my breathing, finding the ujjayi breathing technique was most valuable. Both the midwives present commented on the ease and depth of the relaxation I was achieving in between contractions. I was able to visualise the opening of my womb and see each contraction as a positive part of the process. Time vanished, I felt removed from those around me and I remember gazing out of the window towards the mountains and feeling very relaxed and dreamy. It was transition, and at this point and I completely surrendered myself, realising nature was taking over, giving the body time to recover and prepare for the next stage of labour.

I soon felt a slight pressure on the anal area as though I needed to move my bowels and after being examined, I was ready to push as I had completely dilated. I got off the bed and into a squatting position leaning over the bed and found I had an incredible urge to push. I was then supported in a squatting position with Rob supporting me from behind. The contractions were at their peak and I felt in control, but not in control—in the sense that nature and instinct had taken over. My mind and body were working as one following their natural course, the inner strength of this process was

truly amazing. My throat quickly became sore and hoarse with the effort and I was surprised how physically demanding this was, as I was using all my stamina and strength to stay with it.

The midwife placed a mirror so I could watch the birth, and the sight of Sarah coming into the world is one I will never forget. When she was born she looked surprised laying on her back, arms and legs spread open, obviously wondering what on earth was happening. I couldn't take my eyes off her and Rob cut the cord.

The first touch, the first cuddle, no words can ever describe the awe of this moment. Time seemed to have stopped and I was lost in a state of disbelief gazing at Sarah, before realising I had the daughter I hardly dared to dream of, for wanting too much. She was soon in Rob's arms, a very special time for both of them as they looked at each other for the first time, becoming completely absorbed in one another. We then spent wonderful hours enjoying ourselves snuggling and enjoying the euphoria.

Pregnancy and childbirth have been a truly wonderful experience, one that I feel thankful to have enjoyed. Although it has offered various challenges, none have been as great or demanding as those that are faced now as a new mother, nor as rewarding. Motherhood adds a new dimension to the word 'Love'.

For anyone reading this who is preparing for labour and birth, I could not recommend strongly enough the practice

of yoga. It can help you with so many aspects of pregnancy, labour and birth, everything from breathing, relaxation, mental approach, physical suppleness, strength and stamina. It has been, and still is invaluable to me.

Jessica Reilly: Pregnancy, Birth and Yoga

I decided to begin yoga classes during the second trimester of my pregnancy and I found it to be so valuable in many ways. So why did I decide to try yoga classes during pregnancy?

There were a number of reasons for this decision. Firstly, my husband was trying to get me to learn to relax after years of stress, poor eating habits and lack of exercise while I was working as a pharmaceutical sales representative and then another short stint back in the classroom in my previous role of a secondary science teacher. I found it difficult to relax and would often find myself clenching my teeth as I slept. I was also taking short rapid breaths while sleeping, and waking up in the morning not feeling refreshed from sleep, even though I may have slept for 7-8 hours. I realised that for my own sake and also my unborn child's I really needed to rectify this problem. The solution was to try yoga to learn to relax and breathe correctly. There was an added benefit in the stretching exercises, which helped to improve my suppleness in preparation for the birth. This led me to Theresa's classes.

CHAPTER 21: Birth stories

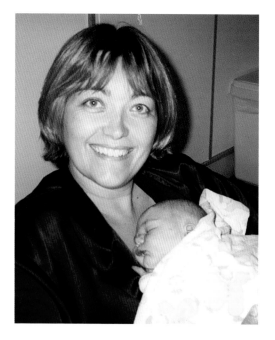

These classes differed from those I had done at the gym in that the exercises and breathing techniques were all aimed at the pregnant woman and her requirements. I found them much easier and finally felt I had found somewhere, which would help me learn to breathe correctly, not only for the birth, but also for life. I think we all found these classes wonderful, and I am sure we all managed to drop off to sleep on more than one occasion!

The result! My breathing improved, I found myself more relaxed and my husband told me that my breathing at night was much better. I was actually starting to feel as though I had a good night's sleep (as much as you can when you are entering the final stages of pregnancy!) I found that the meditations were the best. My particular favourite was the candle meditation, which would relax me almost instantly and I also found it the easiest to focus on.

How did yoga help me? I went into labour on a Sunday afternoon and had to go to hospital immediately as my waters had broken. I did not use any pain relief at all through the afternoon and night. I was very focused on what I was doing and also used the different breathing techniques I was shown to help me through the contractions as they increased in intensity (ante natal classes do not teach breathing techniques anymore). My husband and I attended the partners' class with Theresa where he was shown some of the breathing and meditation techniques I had been learning, and massage. This proved very beneficial as he helped me (reminded me) what I had learnt and encouraged me to use those breathing techniques. It was unfortunate that the candle could not be used in the labour ward (no open flames are permitted in the hospital rooms), but I did focus on a light, which helped. At 6 a.m. the following morning, I began on the gas, as the contractions were becoming much more intense. Then one and a half hours later there was bedlam in the room as my son was in distress and we had to have an emergency caesarean with a general anaesthetic but I awoke to a very healthy young boy whom we called Loughlin Thomas Reilly.

Loughlin is a very placid and relaxed child. I feel within myself that part of this is because I learnt to relax with the yoga classes during my pregnancy, and I am still using the basic techniques I learnt whenever I become uptight again. There was another bonus to these classes. I met a number of wonderful ladies whom I am still in contact with. We meet on a regular basis and continue the friendship that was begun in the classes. These classes were also an avenue to discuss our pregnancy and discuss our feelings with a group of people who were also going through the same changes in their lives. It was a wonderful support network and I would highly recommend it to any pregnant woman!

These are my birth stories. Without doubt every mother has her own unique birth story, all very different and each a transformation event in her life as a woman. For this reason I have included a special chapter dedicated to personal birth journeys, in which very different women have shared their special moments and thoughts about how yoga played a significant role during pregnancy and in preparation for labour and birth, as well as how valuable the different techniques proved to be after the birth.

CHAPTER 22

THE FIRST TWELVE MONTHS

Care for yourself first and then you can better care for your baby.

Pregnancy, labour and birth are only the beginning of a new and extraordinary part of your life—as a mother. And as natural and normal as that is, it is also a completely unique and unfamiliar situation full of joy and wonder, unexpected challenges and unexplored territory. Apart from the fact that now there is a baby to care for, which is a full-time job in itself, it is also a time of new and bewildering inconsistencies to cope with day by day. This includes the sudden hormonal changes that take place soon after birth, the fluctuating emotions that often accompany them, and extreme fatigue simply because you are dealing with lack of sleep and the newness of it all. Along with this come the predictable over-effort and self-inflicted pressures of trying to be the best mother possible for your new baby, and the realisation that even if you have a supportive partner and family you are no longer 'on your own'. Although this seems self-evident, it can still be quite a shock. All this can take real time to adjust to and is enough to throw a normally very organised life into near chaos.

When you're in the full, glorious bloom of pregnancy, 'life after birth' is a subject that seems too far removed to think about. It's only when you are at home with your baby that you find yourself quite suddenly in one of life's most rewarding but also time-consuming roles—where you are on call physically and emotionally 24 hours of the day.

Most of the time being a new mother is an absolute joy and wonder. But at times you will feel completely overwhelmed and wonder if you will ever be the mother you hoped to be, or even if you will make it to the end of the day. It is a time in your life like no other, when it is particularly important to be gentle and patient with yourself and to make sure you are nourished, so you can nourish in turn. For your wellbeing and that of your baby, you need to be able to accept the enormous changes that have occurred fro being a woman on your own to a new mum, almost overnight.

My intention here is to remind you of what you have already learnt through yoga and to encourage you to use some of the simple skills now, for you will appreciate their value even more than before, and to emphasise—take it easy, go slowly, keep your expectations realistic and attainable. The only way to learn about mothering and what life is like with your newborn is to live it and to move as gently as possible through each moment. Live one day at a time consciously and mindfully, as you did during your pregnancy and take extra

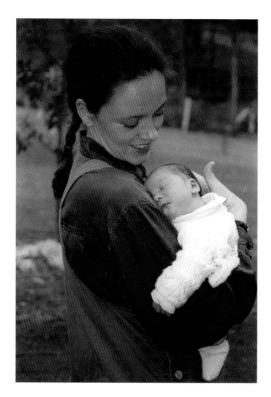

more than one level, just as your whole life has. Your hormones are adjusting to normal again. For some women the 'three-day blues' that occur naturally after the birth can linger many days longer than that, with an emotional intensity that can be quite unexpected.

As well as these physical and emotional changes you are also dealing with the fact that you now have not only your own life and your partner's to consider, but your tiny baby's too. Your baby's whole world is you and she is dependant on you totally—which means at any time of day or night, regardless of whether you are tired, need to prepare dinner, making an attempt to tackle the week's ironing. So it is important not to become distressed when things just aren't getting done right now, to realise that life does eventually sort itself out.

Despite the difficulties this is of course a truly joyous time with beautiful, beautiful moments that you will hold forever in your heart. It is my intention to reflect on the reality of motherhood, both glorious and difficult, where euphoria coexists with the general chaos and disorder of early parenting. Being a mother is instinctive and intuitive, so go quietly with your feelings, relax a lot and most of all enjoy—with a little help from your partner, family and friends, and your knowledge of yoga.

By being aware and more realistically informed, the heartache and even disillusionment some women feel in their

care of yourself, just as you did then. Remember, to cherish others you must first cherish yourself.

So many women tell me they wish someone had told them how tired and overwhelmed they were going to feel after the birth, how amazed they are that this gorgeous, tiny baby could have turned their whole life upside down within a couple of days. They are bewildered that they can't see their way back to their previous life, facing the realisation that being a mother is a much bigger and tougher job than they were aware of and prepared for. Becoming a new mother is a big deal, and that needs to be acknowledged.

It helps to remember that your body has undergone enormous changes on

new role can be reduced. It is not until you are actually living this new roles along with the roles of woman, wife, cook, family counsellor, cleaner, daughter, friend, etc.—that all those 'at home with your baby' stories you have heard become real. This is where some simple yoga skills can help you enjoy and relax into these precious days even more and live your life moment to precious moment.

It is especially important now to take some time for yourself to simply relax and be present, because how you look after yourself physically and emotionally will impact on how you cope day to day.

Many women find the yoga skills they learnt during pregnancy are even more valuable after the birth, some even using them instinctively when they were needed the most. Conscious breath awareness is always there to help you bring your mind back to yourself, and the breathing exercises will help you feel calm and relaxed, just as they did before. As little as five minutes is all you need to rest in the quiet space of your mind. It will help immensely to restore your energies and balance—an inbuilt survival skill.

Deep Relaxation

In the months after the birth you might still be feeling quite tired, at times even exhausted, both physically and emotionally. While some women feel quite well quite quickly, others take a lot longer to feel themselves again. There is no point comparing yourself with other new mothers. How you feel is influenced by numerous things—how much sleep you are getting and how easily your baby has settled into life, for example. When your baby is sleeping take the opportunity, as often as possible, to take a rest yourself to recharge your batteries and restore strength and balance. When you do this you will find your time with your baby much more enjoyable, and a lot easier too. I know there are always too many jobs to be done while baby sleeps, and it is true that women will always find something that needs doing. But I'll say it again—the more you care and nourish yourself the better you will care for your baby.

Every day remember to do some slow, deep breathing to restore your energy, consciously breathing in the qualities and feelings you most want for yourself. It takes so little time and does wonders for mind and body. If you need to release fatigue or tension, the deep cleansing breaths are there to help you relax. The Candle Meditation is very useful now—it is a wonderful way to stop for a moment, to be still, and reflect on what life has brought you.

Humming and Ujjayi Breathing

Many women have used humming after the birth for its calming effects on them and on their babies. Using a soft humming breath to relax while breast-feeding can help settle a baby. If your baby is restless or distressed rest her on your chest and hum softly. She will hear the sound and

often be calmed—maybe remembering the healing sound and soothing vibrations from the womb. Humming will often quieten a baby and help her sleep soundly, even many months after the birth.

Humming gently while rocking your baby in your arms is a wonderful opportunity to connect with each other, mother and baby. Such precious moments are both timeless and transient—enjoy being absorbed in each other in the quiet and peaceful space that gentle humming gives you.

Tanya came to yoga for her pregnancies. She enjoyed humming then, and it is still in her life many years later:

One of the most precious gifts I gave my two babies was yoga as it provided me with so many benefits during pregnancy, in labour and as a new mother. The humming was one my favourites as I found it very calming and peaceful—its vibrations through my body helped me centre and relax. When my first son Corey was six weeks old to my surprise he started humming to himself, often before sleeping … I'm sure he remembered it from being in my womb. He is five now and still hums when we cuddle, it is our special time to reconnect through this healing sound.

The relaxing ujjayi breathing exercise is a valuable life skill that you might find yourself intuitively using after the birth and for many years ahead. When you were pregnant your baby could hear you breathing and feel the calmness the

throat breath gave you, which meant the atmosphere in the womb would also have been peaceful. Vivian told me she used ujjayi breathing to calm her baby Camille whenever she was restless, holding her to her chest, close to her throat. Camille always relaxed very quickly and slept very soundly afterward.

After your baby has finished feeding spend a little time resting with her on your chest, gently humming or doing ujjayi breathing. This is a beautiful way to end this special time together, and to embrace these brief moments.

Taking care of your own wellbeing will mean you, and your baby, are much happier and contented and life will flow more smoothly. Reflect on the changes that have occurred so quickly in your life, in less than a year, and acknowledge how well you have done in these early days of mothering—and simply appreciate yourself.

Postnatal Exercise and Yoga Programs

The postnatal exercise and yoga program detailed here will not be suitable for every woman, as personal wellbeing, and your baby's health and temperament, will all have a bearing on whether you are ready—or even interested—in taking up yoga again soon after the birth. If you are having an easy time feeding your baby and she has settled well, you will be more likely to consider doing some gentle exercises than if she is colicky, say, and your sleep pattern is completely disrupted.

I have outlined a balanced, easy to manage program which can be integrated into your day by spending a little time on it, whenever it is appropriate, in the comfort of your own home. Many of the exercises can be done while watching TV or sitting in the garden under a shady tree with your baby.

Don't be hard on yourself when contemplating an exercise program. Your body has just undergone some massive changes physically and emotionally, and your hormones are slowly adjusting to normal again. Be gentle with yourself and realise that you will regain your shape and figure over time. Don't panic when your favourite clothes don't fit in the first weeks and even months after the birth. It's a fact of life that some women return to their pre-pregnancy shape more quickly than others, but that's because we are all unique and all made differently.

The First Six Weeks

Your time and attention will at first be completely involved in caring for your newborn and exploring the joy and wonder of being a mother. In the early days of your baby's life, close bonds and spiritual relationships are formed between you, your child and your partner which last a lifetime. This is a precious and very transient time as you come to know your baby's unique personality.

During this time it is very important to ensure your own needs are not neglected. Have plenty of rest, eat nourishing foods and drink plenty of fluids, especially if you are breast-feeding. It is not advisable to begin exercises or postures until the lochia (after-birth bleeding) has completely ceased. However, you can resume deep relaxation, breathing exercises and meditation as soon after the birth as you wish. They will assist in restoring balance and harmony on all levels and help to

replenish your energies. I strongly advise taking up the pelvic floor exercises soon after the birth to return firmness and strength to your perineum and pelvic floor muscles.

If the birth was reasonably straightforward, it is quite acceptable to include a few gentle head lifts, to restore tone and fitness to your abdominal area. These are best done lying on your back with your knees bent. Do them slowly and without effort, between five and ten each day. If you had an exhausting labour, however, more time will be needed for recovery. As a general rule always ask your doctor or midwife before proceeding.

Any yoga stretching exercises should be avoided until at least six to eight weeks after the birth, and fitness programs or strenuous exercises should be postponed for a lot longer. If you had a caesarean

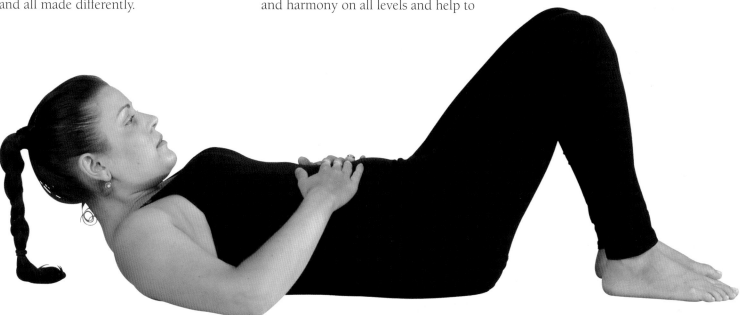

delivery, do not begin any exercises until you have your doctor's approval. One woman who came to yoga throughout her pregnancy and had a caesarean delivery told me it was almost six months to the day before she felt completely at ease with her normal yoga program, even though she was yoga fit before the birth and began classes again when her baby was about nine weeks old.

Six Weeks After the Birth

By the time your baby is six weeks old you may feel like beginning some gentle yoga exercises. The exercises suggested here will restore tone and flexibility, and remove any stiffness you might be feeling. Approach your yoga with a quiet mind and gentle attitude and do just a little at a time. You will be happier and more relaxed, and this state of being will help your baby to stay calm and relaxed too.

The benefits of resuming a simple yoga and exercise program after the birth include encouraging your pelvic floor muscles and perineum to become firm and strong, and the muscles of your uterus to return to normal size. Your back is kept supple and flexible, the spinal column and spinal nerves are nourished and strengthened, helping to relieve tension in your neck and back muscles. Your abdominal muscles are firmed and toned and your circulation improved. If you can find a little time each day to rest, relax and possibly do a short meditation you will find your energy levels improve and you

are less fatigued—and you will survive lack of sleep better.

I suggest you only include these gentle exercises and concentrate more on relaxation and the breathing exercises. Spending time in the Child Pose will give you the same relaxation that it did while you were pregnant, and stretch gently into your back. Exercises for the hands, the shoulders and the neck will alleviate tension in the upper body especially if your back is tight and if you are feeling exhausted. The Cat can be included now and pelvic rocking, and some gentle rocking from side to side on your back with the knees in to the chest. Some women enjoy the Mountain at this time to relieve tightness in the back and legs— either the full posture or the variation leaning against the wall. If you enjoyed the balancing postures, I would add the Tree, the easy Standing Spinal Twist (page 70) and the easy seated spinal twists (page 58). Whatever you choose to do, always start by loosening your body first, and finish with some breathing exercises and deep relaxation.

> **Caution:** At no time are the exercises meant to cause strain or result in fatigue. Begin slowly with the simpler stretches and postures and approach them in such a way as to nurture and fulfil your needs rather than as a workout program.

Eight to Twelve Weeks After the Birth

If you are feeling well and strong around this time and have your doctor's approval, you might like to add the postures listed here to your six-week routine, including the single leg lifts.

The Heavenly Stretch (page 69) can be included now, and the other seated spinal twists modified for pregnancy. The Triangle Side Bend (page 71) will feel good, giving its lovely stretch through the side of your body. The modified Wide-A Leg Stretch (page 76) can be included also. By completing a forward bend, a spinal twist and a side bend, you are working the spinal column in all directions. All these exercises are simple and safe to do unless you are experiencing back problems or have been advised against them.

Single Leg Lift Lying on Your Back

This exercise is excellent for toning your abdominal muscles and thighs but it important to take things slowly, as the abdominal muscles take time to regain their original firmness. At no time continue the exercise if you feel strain in the abdominal area, or if your breathing becomes short and tense.

Keep one leg bent with your foot on the floor. As you inhale the other leg is slowly lifted as high as you can take it. Exhale as the leg is lowered to the floor. Although keeping one leg bent reduces the impact of the exercise, it is the safest way

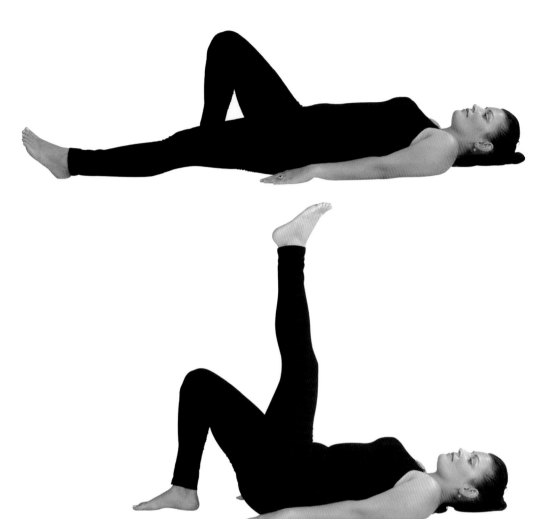

remembering always that the time you are spending doing yoga should be enjoyable. As always, remember the pelvic floor exercises every day and the value of time in relaxation to restore your energies.

The exercises are suggested as a general guide, providing they are helping you and making you feel good. Always listen to your body and do what is best for you, moving along quietly at your own pace. The dangers of not listening to your body and ignoring early warning signs such as painful muscles and fatigue could, over time, lead to a decreased milk supply, sleep disorders or moodiness, depression and irritability. When the body's signals are completely ignored, it becomes exhausted and more serious conditions can develop.

You can approach the yoga postures almost as a meditation in motion, feeling yourself moving from one posture to the next as your breath and your movements are unified—always witnessing your inner self and the flow of energy and prana deep within you. You will notice a profound sense of grace and stillness when yoga is practised in this way.

Now you can also include the other balancing and triangle postures (pages 80 and 71) and the seated Wide Leg Stretch (page 31). All the seated spinal twists can be done, as well as those practiced lying on your back. And allow some time at the end of your program for the breathing exercises, meditation and deep relaxation.

to approach it. Repeat five lifts with each leg, then gently rock your body from side to side with your knees held close to your chest. Always flatten the middle of your back by pressing it to the floor, so you are using your abdominal muscles rather than your back muscles to lift your leg. This is also a safeguard against straining your back. Some women find it helpful to place their hands—palms down—under their hips when practising the leg lifts and any of the other abdominal exercises, as

this encourages the back to stay flat on the floor instead of arching.

Twelve Weeks After the Birth

When your baby is around twelve weeks old, your life will have settled considerably and you might have more energy and a little more time for yourself. You can now include a number of exercises to those you are already practising to make a complete mini yoga program of your own. Choose the postures that best suit your needs,

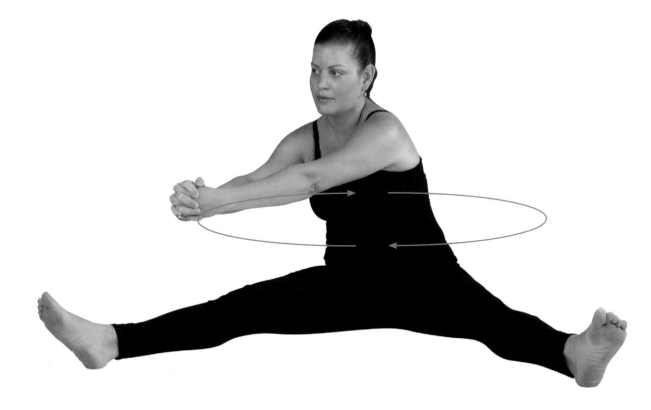

Seated Wide Leg Stretch and Churning the Mill

Prepare for Churning the Mill as you did while you were pregnant (see page 33).

Now, however, you can extend back much further than before, working more deeply into your abdominal area. Do not lean right back to the floor as you swing through the semi-circular movement, but just enough to feel your abdominal muscles working. If you go too close to the floor, returning to the upright position can strain your lower back muscles. You might find it more comfortable to sit on a cushion for this and the next exercise.

Rowing the Boat

This exercise will give a good stretch to
your hamstring muscles at the back of
your legs and also tone your abdominals.

1. Sit with your legs to the front and
   your feet together, using a cushion if
   necessary. Stretch your arms out to the
   front and join your hands.
2. Breathe in to prepare and breathe out
   as you stretch forward over both legs,
   feeling the stretch in the back of your
   legs. Breathe in and lean back as you
   bring the hands into the chest, as if you
   were rowing a boat, then breathe out
   as you lean forward. Continue to do
   this as many times as you wish. This
   can be included after the exercises for
   your feet and the hip rotations from the
   pregnancy program and as part of the
   abdominal exercises.

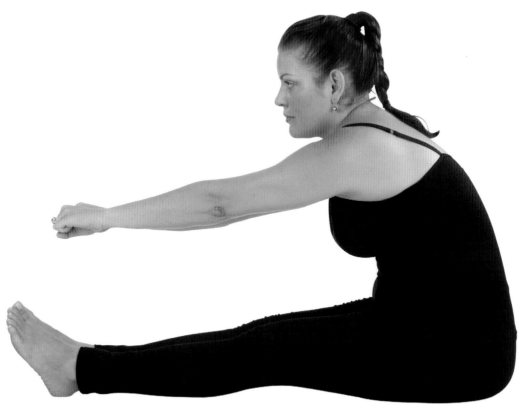

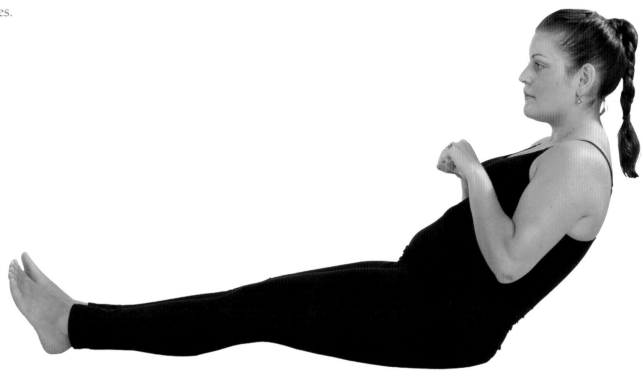

The Head to Knee Pose:
Janu Sirshasana

The Head to Knee pose was not included during pregnancy as many women find it quite uncomfortable, but as a postnatal exercise it offers many benefits. It increases flexibility in your hips and stretches deeply throughout the muscles of your back and hamstrings. This stretch tones and gently massages the abdominal organs, and reduces excess fat from that part of the body. It is recommended for the health of the reproductive system, and highly recommended for women who suffer menstrual difficulties. This posture also relaxes deeply into the mind, another benefit of the head-down position. The longer you relax into the forward bend the more you will stretch the body and feel a wonderful calm response in the mind. It is important not to over-extend in the final position, remaining relaxed at all times.

1. Sit with your back straight, on a cushion for extra lift in your pelvis and for comfort.
2. Bend your right leg and place your right foot beside your left inner thigh.
3. Breathe in to prepare and breathe out and move into the stretch over your left leg. Although the aim is to have your head resting on your knee, it is more important to come only as far forward as you can in complete comfort—never push yourself beyond where you can relax into the final position. Practiced in this way, all the benefits, mental and physical will be enjoyed, wherever you find yourself in the final position. Even with continued practice some people find it difficult to reach the full extension, either due to injury or simply because of the way they are made. Once you are in the full stretch, close your eyes, relax and breathe into the stretch. This can be held for nine breaths or more; the longer you remain the more you will ease into the stretch and the more relaxed your mind will be.
4. Breathe in to come up and repeat the stretch with the other leg to the front.

Always do some pelvic rocking on the hands and knees and then rest in the Child Pose when you have completed the posture, or rest on your back with your knees held into your chest rocking from side to side.

This is quite an adequate group of postures to add now. Unless you have a personal desire or need to do something more strenuous and demanding, I would continue with this program until your baby is at least five or six months old.

> **Note:** This posture is not suitable for people with severe back problems such as a slipped disc.

Six Months After the Birth

When your baby is six months old it is safe to include all the exercises and postures recommended for pregnancy.

I suggest including Salute to the Sun (page 212), after doing some light stretching, and before the other postures. A number of other excellent asanas are also appropriate at this time, as they have particular relevance for balancing the female reproductive system. This is a comprehensive group of asanas, but still only a small section of the thousands that are available. It is also worth noting that all of these postures are ideal for women throughout their lives, from pre-puberty to after menopause.

As always, before commencing these postures choose a selection of other exercises and postures that complement those detailed here.

In the next chapter I outline six programs which include these new postures.

Note: If your baby was born by caesarean section I do not recommend these postures be considered until at least six months, and after you have consulted your medical professionals.

The Boat: *Naukasana*

The Boat is a quite strenuous posture that works deeply into your abdominal muscles. Never strain, quiver or repeat the exercise so often that you end up with sore muscles for days afterward. If you consider that you were pregnant for nine months and your baby is only five or six months old now, it is reasonable to assume that these muscles are still a little weak and need to be treated with respect. It is better to gradually increase the number over time, so that muscle tone and strength can be developed progressively. I suggest you practise this after Rowing the Boat (page 197) and the Single Leg Lift for a complete mini-abdominal program.

It is important to elevate your legs and body to an equal height. Experiment a little, lifting your legs and body higher or lower, until you eventually find the most balanced and also most demanding position.

You will immediately notice the benefits to your abdominal area as tone, strength and firmness are improved. The function of your digestive system is enhanced and regular practise of this posture will bring balance to your nervous system. Your back muscles will be strengthened, which is particularly important as it is often strained or weakened during pregnancy.

1. Lie on your back with your body straight and relaxed.
2. Breathe in as you lift your head, shoulders, arms, feet and legs from the floor, keeping your legs the same height as your head and shoulders. Stretch through your arms and point the fingers towards your toes. You will resemble a wide V, lifting up about 30 centimetres off the floor.
3. Breathe out as you lower your body to the floor.
4. Repeat this up to five times.
5. Rest and relax when you have completed the practice. You might like to bring the knees into the chest and rock gently from side to side.

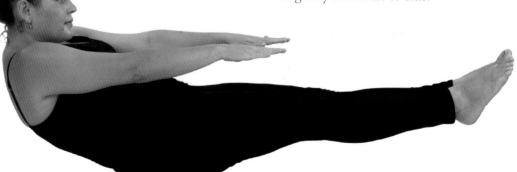

Note: The following four postures—the Plough Preparation, the Half Shoulder Stand, the Shoulder Stand and the Plough—can be grouped together as their benefits overlap and they are often practised in sequence. They are usually attempted under the supervision of a teacher, but if the instructions and precautions are followed carefully there is no reason why they cannot be learnt from my book. It is a matter of taking complete responsibility for what you do and how you are doing it, so that the benefits and rewards can be enjoyed to their fullest.

Note: It is important to always keep your head still in the final postures and come out of the postures very slowly. These postures are best approached slowly and always with a responsible awareness.

Caution: These postures are not recommended for people with spinal problems, slipped discs, cardiac and blood pressure disorders. There is also a caution for people suffering thyroid gland dysfunction, who should not consider doing them unless you have been given the approval of your doctor and are under the care of a teacher who has a thorough understanding of your medical condition. In the case of mild thyroid insufficiency I would only recommend the Plough Preparation posture.

It is preferable to practise these asanas on an empty stomach, or at least three hours after a meal and it is very important to warm up first. They are usually done at the end of the exercise section of a yoga program, which should include Salute to the Sun—this way your body is loose and relaxed.

In general, the head-down postures supply your brain with a rich blood flow, improving concentration and sharpening your memory, while relieving pressure and tiredness in your feet and legs. When the body is returned to the prone position, the lower limbs receive a nourishing supply of blood, the position overall resulting in balance and rejuvenation of your whole being.

The major organs of your digestive system and pelvic region , are relieved of pressure which is useful for conditions such as prolapse, constipation and diverticulitis. Your glandular system is revitalised and your nervous system balanced and strengthened.

When first attempting this group of postures, I would advise holding the final posture for only five breaths at a time and extending that gradually after regular practice.

The Plough Preparation:
Poorwa Halasana

The Plough Preparation is a safe and easy preparation for the Plough and the Shoulder Stand. Be very aware of how you are feeling in this posture and don't proceed to the more advanced postures until you feel completely at ease. If you want more lift in your pelvis, a small folded blanket or a few cushions can be placed under your hips for a greater tilt. This posture is practised with your buttocks close to a wall and your feet resting against the wall and your legs slightly bent. Until you are completely relaxed and confident in the Half and Full Shoulder stands I would always suggest you approach them from this position for extra support and safety. When your legs are in this position they can be taken off the wall and replaced when you need to. It is not uncommon for people to find the Shoulder Stand and Plough too uncomfortable and to prefer this supported variation, which still supplies all the benefits of the more difficult postures.

1. Lie on your back with your buttocks close to the wall. Bend your knees and place your feet on the wall. Place your hands in a tight fist under your buttocks or, for a greater tilt, place cushions under your buttocks. Your head, shoulders and the middle of your back remain on the floor throughout this exercise. Some people like to

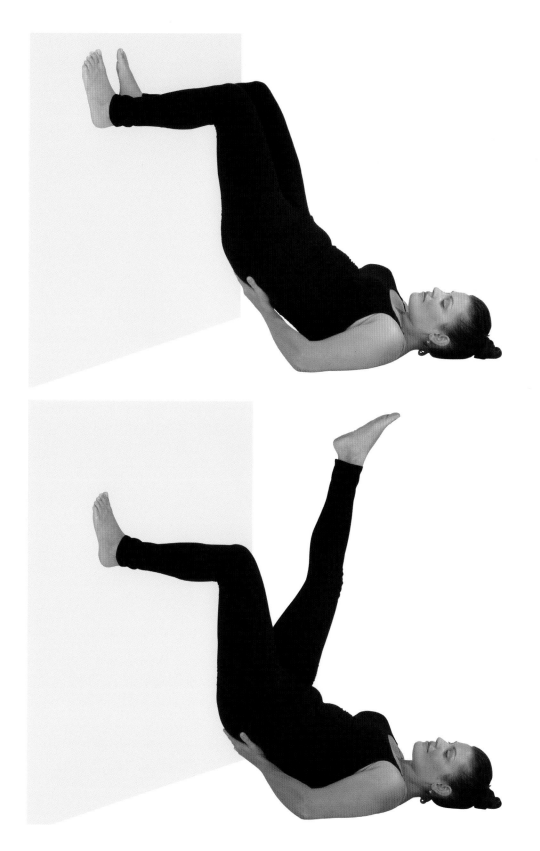

pause in this position and adjust to the feeling before proceeding.

2. When you are ready, lift your hips a little higher and hold that posture while you breathe and relax. This is really a supported Shoulder Stand and might be as far as you want to go until you become familiar with the position. The feet can be walked up the wall as you elevate your hips higher, but I suggest you keep your knees bent rather than straightening your legs.

3. If this posture is comfortable and there is no feeling of fullness in your face you can lift your hips higher and feel your chin a little closer to your upper chest. Remember to adjust your position to best suit your needs at the time. Your legs are still slightly bent with your feet flat on the wall. Your back is not straight here and you should feel no breathlessness or pressure on the chest or fullness in your face. If you do experience any discomfort, lower yourself a little until you are completely comfortable.

4. With your hips supported, ease your right leg towards your face, holding this for a short time before returning your leg to the wall. Repeat this with the left leg. These movements can be repeated as often as you like or held for a short time while breathing quietly. When you are confident your legs can be taken off the wall together, briefly, for the Half Shoulder Stand. At this point it might be more comfortable to

bring the elbows a little closer together. When your feet are taken away from the wall, your shoulders and upper body take the full weight of your lower body, which is why it is important to proceed very slowly with the exercise. Rest from this position by putting your feet back on the wall.

5. When you are ready to come out of the posture, lower your hips to the floor and rest on your back, and remove your hands or cushions from under your hips. Rest and relax now, preferably with your knees bent to your chest, and gently rock from side to side before sitting up.

Any discomfort in your lower back after completing this posture and the next one will be quickly relieved by this gentle rocking, or by resting in the Child Pose.

The Half Shoulder Stand:
Viipareetakarani Asana
There are many important benefits for the whole internal body from practising the Half Shoulder Stand and the Full Shoulder Stand, primarily because the inverted position of the body reverses the effects of gravity:

• The digestive system is revitalised, resulting in improved health and better organ function. This means that the stomach and the bowel will operate more efficiently.

• Constipation and haemorrhoids can be relieved with continued practice, and minor disorders of the small and large intestine remedied. This has particular relevance for those suffering with diverticulitis or pockets in the bowel that cause pain, bloating and discomfort. When the bowel works more efficiently, harmful toxins are removed from the body, resulting in feelings of increased wellbeing and good health. If there is a predisposition to prolapse of the uterus and bowel, practising these postures is an ideal way of preventing the problem becoming worse.

• Taking the weight off the muscles of the pelvic floor plays an important role in overcoming any weakness in that part of the body. This is especially true in the event of mild incontinence,

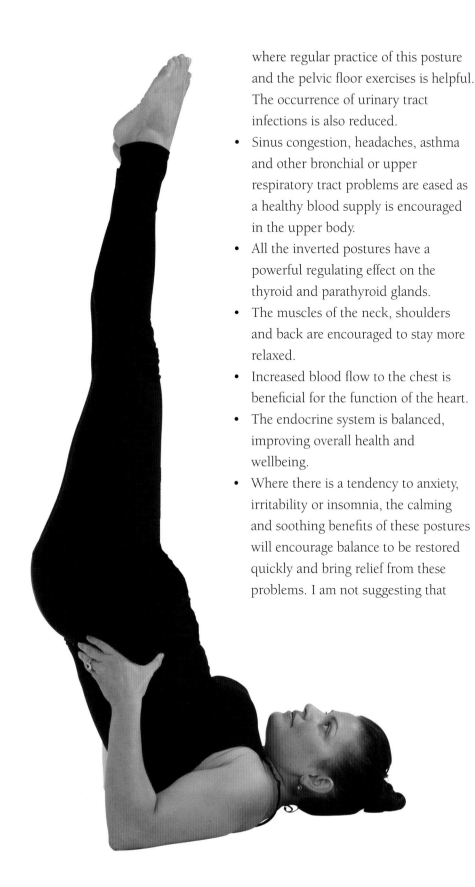

where regular practice of this posture and the pelvic floor exercises is helpful. The occurrence of urinary tract infections is also reduced.

- Sinus congestion, headaches, asthma and other bronchial or upper respiratory tract problems are eased as a healthy blood supply is encouraged in the upper body.
- All the inverted postures have a powerful regulating effect on the thyroid and parathyroid glands.
- The muscles of the neck, shoulders and back are encouraged to stay more relaxed.
- Increased blood flow to the chest is beneficial for the function of the heart.
- The endocrine system is balanced, improving overall health and wellbeing.
- Where there is a tendency to anxiety, irritability or insomnia, the calming and soothing benefits of these postures will encourage balance to be restored quickly and bring relief from these problems. I am not suggesting that

by simply practising the inverted postures all emotionally-related disorders will be alleviated, but with continued and regular practice in conjunction with breathing, meditation and other therapies, the problems will definitely be reduced over time and balance restored to the whole person. Yoga works very deeply and effectively on the internal body and when the endocrine system and the nervous systems are balanced many emotionally-related problems can be reduced.

- These excellent postures are specific for restoring and maintaining optimum health in the female reproductive system. They are designed to create tone and strength in the body while superior function is established to the reproductive organs, relevant to women of all ages.

In the Half Shoulder Stand your body is held at a 45 degree angle with your eyes in line with your toes. It is important, in the beginning, to be aware of any shortness of breath, restricted breathing or excessive fullness in your face. If any of these symptoms bother you, it would be better to more time in the Plough Preparation before trying again. I don't recommend practising the Full Shoulder Stand until you feel completely relaxed and safe in the Half Shoulder Stand.

When you first practice this posture and the Full Shoulder Stand I suggest doing them with your feet resting on the wall for safety. Some people like to place a small piece of foam or thin blanket under the neck for extra support.

1. Begin by lying on your back with your body straight and relaxed. Rest your hands beside your body and breathe regularly.
2. Bend your knees and bring your legs close in to your chest. Place your hands under your hips to support your back. Keep your elbows parallel to your body rather than out to the sides.
3. Lift your hips away from the floor and, keeping your elbows on the floor, balance your hips on your hands so that they are taking the weight of your body. Relax into this position before proceeding. Keep your breathing even and steady.
4. Elevate your legs to a position where your toes are in line with your eyes and your body is 45 degrees off the ground rather than straight up. Keep your hands under your hips. Do not turn your head when you are in the posture or as you come out of it. This

can be held while you are relaxed and breathing evenly.

5. Come out of the posture slowly and steadily, taking two breaths to return to the floor. Take a final inhalation in the full posture and, while exhaling, lower your back gently to the floor with your hands supporting your back. Your legs will now be upright and your back flat on the floor. From there, take another inhalation and, as you breathe out, either lower your legs to the floor or bend your legs and bring them into your chest. When you lower your legs to the floor your hands can be placed under your buttocks to alleviate back strain and prevent the middle of your back from arching. Bend your knees with your feet flat on the floor if you experience any discomfort in your lower back. Coming out of the Half Shoulder Stand in this way gives you much more control over your movements and reduces the chance of injury.
6. A suitable counter-pose can now be practised.

The Full Shoulder Stand: *Sarvangasana*

This posture is often known as the mother of all yoga postures. The Sanskrit word *sarvanga* means 'whole body', and the practice of *sarvangasana* involves your entire body. Approach this posture with care and a sensible attitude, with awareness of how you are feeling during and after the practice.

1. Follow positions 1 to 3 of the Half Shoulder Stand.
2. When you are ready, straighten your legs and body so that you are completely erect with your hands firmly supporting the middle of your back. Your body and legs should be in line and your chin pressed against the centre of your chest.
3. Breathe regularly, in a quiet and easy manner. Keep your body relaxed and steady and as still as possible. It is very important not to turn your head but to keep it still throughout the whole practice and as you return to the floor.
4. If you are new to the Shoulder Stand, hold the posture for only one or two minutes or even less if that seems too long. With practice, this time can be extended for as long as you are relaxed and comfortable.
5. Follow procedures 5 and 6 of the Half Shoulder Stand to come out of the posture and relax.

Caution: While this posture usually works very well for those suffering from stiffness or tension in the neck, it can occasionally aggravate the situation.

Note: When the inverted postures are completed, always practise a counter-pose such as the Pelvic Tilt or the Shoulder pose (see page 210), the Cat or the Tiger, and finally the Child Pose.

The Plough: *Halasana*

The Plough is the final inverted posture covered in this chapter. It is traditionally practised following the Shoulder Stand and before moving into a counter-pose. The Sanskrit word *hala* means 'plough'. In the final posture your body resembles a traditional hand plough. The middle of your body is contracted so your whole abdominal area is greatly stimulated and massaged. Intestinal gas and bloating are relieved, and disorders or minor upsets to your digestive system are eliminated. Your spinal column and the muscles of your back and the backs of your legs are stretched and you will feel a wonderful stretch in these parts of the body.

1. Begin in the Half Shoulder Stand or the Shoulder Stand. Keeping your legs straight, lower your legs over your head until your toes are touching the floor behind your head. If you are unable to reach the floor with your toes, cushions or a low stool can be placed so that your toes can rest on them instead of over extending towards the floor. You could also place yourself so that your toes come to rest on the seat of a couch or on a step.

2. Extend out into the full Plough in your own time. It is also easier to do if your feet are slightly apart rather than together, and your knees are slightly bent. A reasonable amount of flexibility is required in your back muscles and hamstrings, so take care to extend only as far as your level of flexibility allows. Your hands support the middle of your back when you first practise this pose. In time the arms can be extended away from your body along the floor and eventually, if you are confident, your arms can be extended in the other directions so that your hands touch your toes.

3. Breathe quietly in the final posture. Relax and be as comfortable as possible. For a more complete Plough, walk your feet away further from your body. This gives a dramatic 'chin lock' and has a positive effect on your thyroid gland.

4. When you want to come out of the posture, always support your back with your hands and return slowly to the floor as for the Shoulder Stand.

5. Lie with your knees tucked into your chest and gently massage your back by rocking slowly from side to side, followed with a counter-pose such as the Pelvic Tilt, the Shoulder Pose and finally the Child Pose.

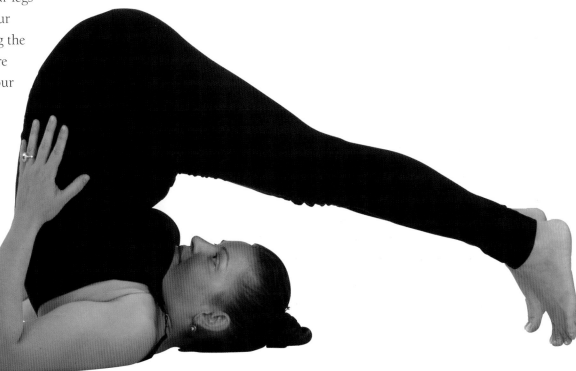

The Dynamic Plough:
Drutahalasana

This wonderfully invigorating exercise is a combination of two postures, the Seated Forward Bend and the Plough. It is a very powerful exercise, and as the name suggests dynamically tones and stimulates your body and brings greater alertness to your mind. I do not recommend this exercise unless you are reasonably fit, as you might find it exhausting rather than stimulating.

The Dynamic Plough is a complete exercise in itself and the whole body is stretched and toned.

> **Caution:** Before commencing the Dynamic Plough, be aware of the precautions and contraindications for the Plough and the Seated Forward Bend (page 198). Do not practise either of the Dynamic Plough variations if you have any back or neck injuries or if you are unable to easily and comfortably perform them.

- You will notice all stiffness, tension and fatigue are removed as you become more supple and flexible in your movements.
- The respiration and heart rate are increased with continued practice, making this an extremely beneficial exercise for the cardiovascular system.

- The back and spinal column are well exercised and massaged due to the rolling movement from the tail bone through to the vertebrae in the neck. This has an invigorating effect on the nervous system, enhancing wellbeing and vitality in the whole body.
- The digestive system is toned and balanced, bringing relief to those suffering with intestinal disturbances such as constipation and diarrhoea. It is also highly recommended for disorders of the liver, gallbladder, stomach and bowel because it has a regulating and rejuvenating effect on those organs. It is an excellent posture for women, especially from six months after the birth.
- The kidneys and adrenal glands are nourished and restored to health, increasing vitality and energy levels.
- This posture will also improve body tone and remove fat deposits, particularly around the waist and hips.

Variation 1

1. Sit on the floor with your body straight, your legs in front of you and your arms beside your body.
2. Breathe in, and as you breathe out bend forward over your legs into the forward stretch. Relax your head towards your legs. Your arms and your shoulders should be loose and relaxed and your legs straight.
3. Continue to breathe naturally as you return to the seated position, and continue moving as you lift your legs over your head into the Plough. Your hands can be brought in to support your back or they can be extended over your head to meet your feet. The feet do not need to reach the floor and your legs can be bent.
4. From the Plough posture roll your body back again over your legs and into the forward bend. Continue to move your body forward and back, repeating this five times or more, depending on how you are feeling.

    You will build momentum and a flowing movement as your body rolls forward over your legs and back into the Plough.

5. When this is complete, rest with your body in a relaxation posture until your breathing and heartbeat have returned to normal. Some people like to rest with their knees bent, or rock slowly from side to side with the knees held to the chest.

Variation 2

1. Begin, as for variation 1, with your body in a seated position.

2. Breathe in and stretch your arms up above your head. Keep your shoulders relaxed and your spine straight and tall.

3. Breathe out as you extend your body over your legs into the full head to knee position. Stretch your hands towards your feet and rest your head on your legs.

4. Breathe in and return to the upright position, keeping your arms stretched above your head and your spine straight.

5. Breathe out as your legs are taken back into the Plough and your hands are behind your head touching your toes.

6. Continue on in this manner, always straightening your spine and bringing your arms above your head when inhaling. This is the important difference between the two variations and it is this strong lift at the midway point which makes this variation physically more demanding.

7. To begin with, practise this four or five times. As your strength and general fitness improve you can increase this number. As with all yoga exercises, rest when the posture is completed, continuing on with other postures only when your breathing and heart rate have returned to normal. Rest with the knees into your chest and rock from side to side.

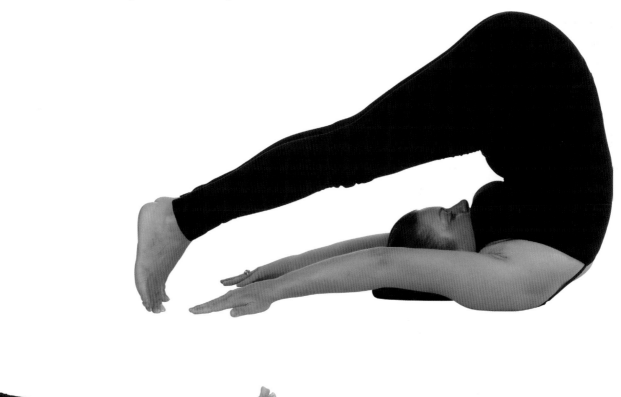

The Sphinx and the Cobra

The Cobra is one of the postures making up the Salute to the Sun. It is an important asana and care needs to be taken when it is practised as a separate posture. The Sphinx is a halfway posture between the floor and the Cobra, and can be practised as a preliminary posture before the Cobra. It is an ideal alternative to the Cobra if you have lower back problems or are extremely stiff in the back.

The benefits of the Sphinx and the Cobra are similar. Your back is arched and made more supple. Circulation to your spine is improved and your spinal nerves are toned. The function and health of the kidneys and adrenal glands greatly benefit from these postures.

As your back is arched and flexed, the front of your body receives a wonderful stretch, especially through the abdominal and pelvic areas, which makes the Cobra one of the most important asanas for the digestive and reproductive systems. The uterus and ovaries are toned, relieving menstrual and gynaecological disorders, while digestion is improved and problems such as mild constipation are alleviated with regular practice. The bladder is also positively affected and rejuvenated with the Cobra.

The Cobra and, to a lesser degree, the Sphinx are specific postures for women and are especially good five or six months after the birth. They are also extremely valuable before conception for optimum health and wellbeing in these parts of the body.

It is important to realise that you will benefit from the Cobra whether you are flexible by nature or not. Always practise within your comfort levels and remember to relax and enjoy the posture. Once you begin to struggle and force yourself into any yoga position, tension is created which then makes it impossible to breathe into the posture and remain relaxed; you also risk injury and soreness.

The Sphinx

1. Prepare by lying on your front with your chin resting on the floor. Rest your lower arms on the floor with your hands flat on the floor beside your face. Keep your legs straight and your feet together, with the upper surfaces of the feet flat on the floor.

2. Breathe in as you lift your upper body as high as possible, keeping your lower arms and your hands on the floor. You might need to adjust the position of your hands so that you can remain in this position in complete comfort. Hold the posture and breathe evenly and gently for five or more breaths. Keep your awareness on your lower back and abdominal area, and relax your body and shoulders.

3. To come out of the Sphinx, breathe out as you lower your body to the floor. This can be repeated three times.

The Cobra: Bhujangasana

In the full Cobra posture you will experience a deep stretch throughout the front of your body from the throat to the navel, and a wonderful arch in the whole of your back. Some people are very flexible in the spine and are able to practise the Cobra effortlessly, whereas others will find they are very stiff in the back and are only able to lift a little higher than in the Sphinx.

1. Prepare as for the Sphinx, then begin to straighten your arms until you have lifted your body off the floor as far as you can without strain or discomfort. It is very important at this point to be completely aware of how you are feeling, never attempting to lift your body higher than you are at ease with. If you find the lift difficult, keep your arms slightly bent or move your hands further apart. With regular practice flexibility will increase and you will be able to lift your body a little higher.

2. Lift your body upright, keep your arms straight, your abdomen and hips on the floor and your shoulders relaxed. If you are completely comfortable in this position and have no neck problems, take your head back for the full Cobra. Remain relaxed, breathing quietly for five breaths, or for as long as you are comfortable. When you first practise the Cobra you might prefer to hold it for two or three breaths, extending the hold as you become more flexible.

3. Lower your body to the floor as you breathe out. This can be repeated three times.

4. On completion rest and relax in the Child Pose, breathing gently.

Caution: If you have a back problem or are recovering from a recent injury practise the Sphinx posture rather than the Cobra. It is a much easier position to manage and will not cause discomfort or strain your back.

The Bow: *Dhanurasana*

The Sanskrit word *dhanu* means 'bow'. In this posture your hands pull on your legs, like a bowstring being tightened to release an arrow. The Bow works in a similar way to the Cobra, where your back is strongly arched and your abdominal area is toned and stretched. The action of your hands on your feet causes your thigh muscles, your abdominal area, and your whole chest and upper back to be worked deeply, while your spinal column is flexed and strengthened. It is an important posture for women of all ages, as the organs of your reproductive system are internally massaged and toned.

Some people find lifting their legs and upper body at the same time quite hard to do. If this is the case, lift your upper body separately from your lower body until you can feel the lift is done easily and in a relaxed manner. It is important to stay relaxed when practising the Bow. Sometimes people try too hard in this exercise, tensing the body in an attempt to obtain the lift, instead of staying relaxed and light. Approach it slowly and without struggle, and in time most difficulties will be overcome.

1. Lie on your front with your legs a little apart, your knees bent and your hands holding onto your feet.
2. Inhale as you lift your legs, chest and head from the floor. Lift your legs and upper body as high as possible. Your pelvic and abdominal areas are the only part of your body remaining on the floor and your arms are straight.
3. Exhale as your body is lowered to the floor. After resting, repeat this up to five times. If you find the Bow easy to do, hold the posture while breathing calmly and regularly. If you are quite flexible in your back and thighs and want a bigger lift, hold onto your ankles instead of your feet.
4. When you have completed the Bow, always relax in the Child Pose.

The Shoulder Pose: *Kandharasana*

The Shoulder pose is very similar in application to the Pelvic Tilt recommended for pregnancy, the difference being that the arch in your back is quite a lot higher. As it has a more dramatic impact on your body than the Pelvic Tilt, it is not recommended for people with abdominal disorders such as peptic ulcers or hernias.

The Shoulder pose has many benefits for your respiratory, digestive and reproductive systems, and is a therapeutic

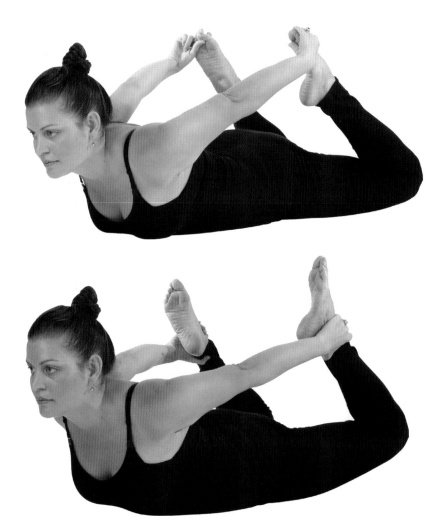

practice for your back and the health of your spinal column. For people suffering from upper respiratory tract disorders, asthma or bronchitis, this is an excellent posture to practise on a regular basis. As with all postures that lock your chin into your chest—such as the Plough and the Shoulder Stand—it is useful for mild thyroid dysfunction. Minor disturbances in your digestive system are corrected and regular function is restored, especially in the colon, stomach and other major organs of that system, due to the position of the body and the full stretch felt in the abdominal area. Regular practice will assist in overcoming such problems as constipation, indigestion and flatulence. The health of your reproductive system is greatly improved making this an excellent posture for women of all ages. The Shoulder pose is an ideal practice for women wanting to conceive, and it is recommended that this posture or the Pelvic Tilt be done soon after intercourse.

The muscles of your back, your spinal column and spinal nerves are all benefited and this is highly recommended for people with constant backache and tight shoulders. This exercise takes the weight off the pelvic floor muscles and is an excellent exercise if you have weakness in that area, preferably combined with regular practice of the pelvic floor exercises and any other postures where your hips are higher than your chest.

1. Lie on your back with your knees bent, your feet hip-distance apart and as close to your buttocks as possible. Rest your arms beside your body and breathe naturally.
2. Lift your hips as high as possible and feel your chin 'locked' close into your chest. Your hands can be placed under your hips to increase the height of the lift, or you can hold onto your ankles if you can reach them. The length of your arms will determine whether you reach your ankles or not—this is related to anatomy rather than degree of flexibility. If you are unable to reach, a piece of thick rope, a strip of fabric or a flat rubber strap can be wrapped around your ankles to make up the difference in arm length. In either of these positions your heels can be lifted off the ground to accentuate the lift.
3. Breathe quietly, holding the posture for five or more breaths.
4. Lower your body to the floor and rest when you have completed the breathing.
5. On completion bring the knees into the chest and rock from side to side.

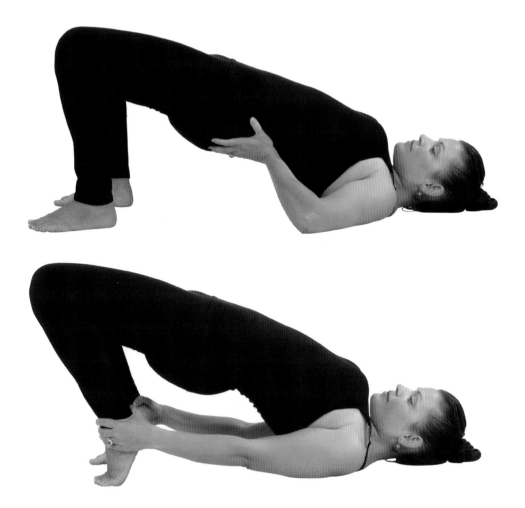

CHAPTER 23

SALUTE TO THE SUN

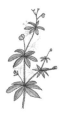

Salute to the Sun, or *surya namskara*, is an excellent way to warm and loosen your body before practising other yoga exercises. It is a sequence of twelve asanas gracefully integrated so that one movement follows the other. Breathing, physical exercise, concentration and awareness are beautifully combined in this flowing expression of yoga. When your body is stretching in one direction, it is simultaneously flexing in the other. The breathing unifies the movements, breathing in for one posture and breathing out for the next, the chest expanding and contracting rhythmically in time with the movements. This results in a greatly increased uptake and utilisation of oxygen and prana in body and mind.

I suggest you begin slowly to familiarise yourself with the way the postures flow and to synchronise your breathing with the movements. Practising slowly also allows you to become more aware of the deep stretch in some of the postures. If it is some time since you have done any physical exercise, you might feel light-headed or breathless when first attempting Salute to the Sun. Although infrequent, dizziness or slight nausea may also be experienced, but through practising slowly and regularly this discomfort will soon go away.

It is up to you how many times you practise this exercise and how quickly or slowly you do it. Some people like to proceed fairly slowly, practising it four or five times with three or four breaths in each position, except position 2 where your arms are above your head. Others choose to do it quite fast, ten times or more, synchronising the movements with the correct breathing. The benefits to the cardiovascular system are greater when the sequence is practised quickly, but the stretch is deeper and more complete if extra time is taken in each position. Practising slowly, however, means you are holding the postures for longer, as you would if they were done on their own, and is more traditional in nature. I find the greatest benefits come from practising the sequence three or four times slowly, then three or four times more quickly.

Generally, the Salute to the Sun can be safely practised by women of all ages and fitness levels, but always be aware of how you are feeling. Rest if you start to feel uncomfortable, then continue at a comfortable pace until your body adjusts to the exercise.

One full round of Salute to the Sun consists of completing the sequence of twelve movements twice. The first time, your right leg is taken back in the Equestrian posture, positions 4 and 10. The second time, take your left leg back. This may differ slightly from other teachings, but I find it the easiest way to remember which leg to take back, and it also helps me keep track of how many rounds I have done.

When you have completed the desired number of rounds, lie on the floor in one of the relaxation positions or the Corpse posture, resting until your heart rate and breathing have stabilised and returned to normal.

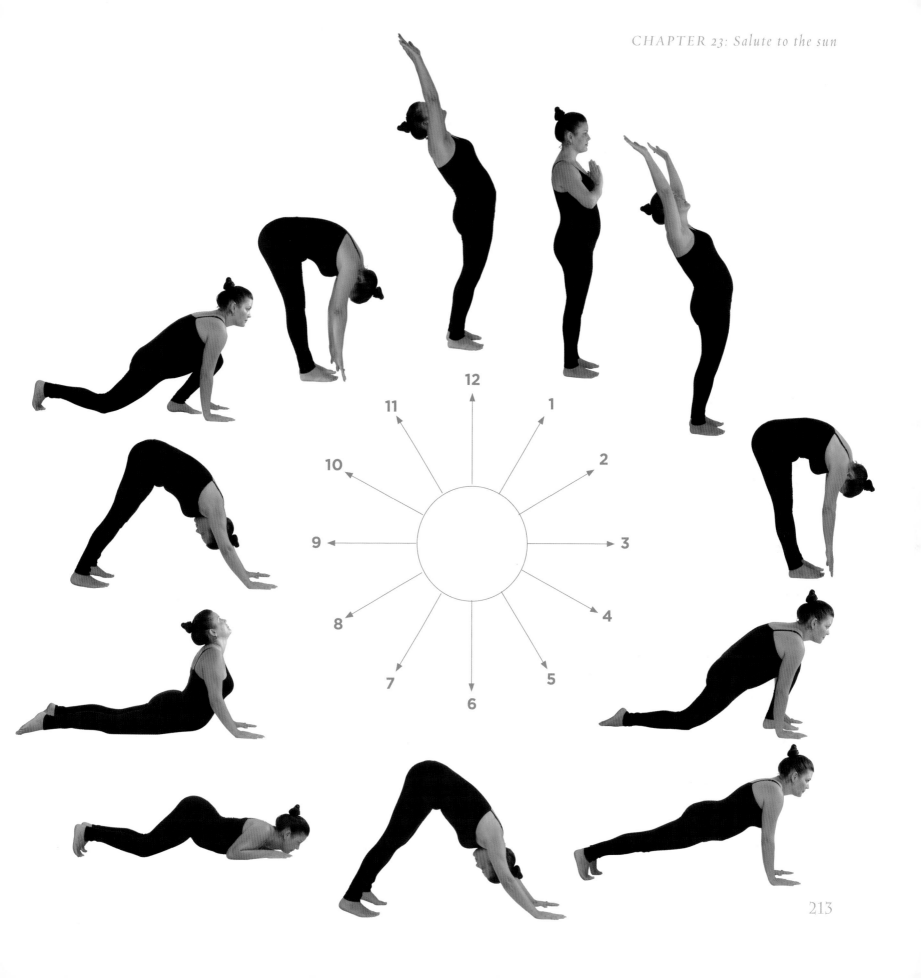

12

11

1

10

2

9

3

8

4

7

5

6

Note: The Salute to the Sun is sometimes taught with slight variations to the sequence detailed here. How you practice it is a personal choice—it is still the Salute to the Sun.

Benefits

- The heart rate is increased, providing quite an aerobic effect. The more often Salute to the Sun is performed, the greater the aerobic effect. It is a dynamic exercise, so take care not to over-extend yourself. It is of the utmost importance to always proceed at your own pace and stop if you feel dizzy or fatigued.

- As respiration is improved due to deeper and more efficient breathing, all the cells of the body are replenished and revitalised with a healthy blood supply and prana. Breathing becomes more efficient as you are enabled to inhale and exhale to a greater capacity and depth, thus increasing the uptake of oxygen and helping remove carbon dioxide. When breathing improves, the lungs can more easily displace and remove the stale air that often remains at the base of the lungs.

- Circulation to all parts of the body is increased. The brain receives a fresh supply of oxygenated blood, bringing freshness to the mind and clarity to the thoughts. Cerebral circulation is improved when your head is down, helping to improve memory, and increase alertness and awareness.

- An enriched blood supply to the digestive system is provided, resulting in improved function and efficiency. Sluggish digestion, constipation, indigestion and many other imbalances of the digestive system can be rectified. The function of all the major organs is improved.

- When respiratory and circulatory systems are working better, the skin receives a greater blood flow. As the skin is one of the major channels of elimination for the body, toxins are more efficiently removed and the skin will glow with health and vitality.

- During the practice of Salute to the Sun, the abdominal organs are alternately stretched and compressed, helping to ensure their optimum function.

- Congestion is removed from the whole body.

- The endocrine system is stimulated and balanced.

- All muscle groups are exercised and toned, bringing relief to stiff muscles. Muscle tension is quickly removed and flexibility is greatly improved.

- Excess fat is removed and the whole body is toned.

- The spine and the central nervous system are nourished and the back muscles toned and strengthened. With regular practice, the spine becomes more supple and flexible, so important to the health and fitness of the whole body.

- The hamstrings and calf muscles are stretched and circulation to the feet and legs is greatly improved.

- With regular practice, mental and physical fatigue are relieved and a much greater sense of balance and wellbeing will be felt throughout the whole body, mind and spirit.

1 The Prayer: *Pranamasana*

Stand with your feet together and your body straight. Join the palms of your hands at the centre of your chest. Feel relaxed and breathe quietly. Before you begin take three deep yoga breaths to become centred and focused.

2 Raised Arms: *Hasta Uttanasana*

Breathe in while raising your arms above your head, arching your body slightly back from the standing position. Stretch deeply throughout your abdominal area, extending through your arms to your fingertips. If you have a very stiff back or are experiencing back problems, stand with your feet further apart and do not extend back as far.

3 Forward Bend: *Padahastasana*

Breathe out and bend your body forward. Stretch your hands towards your feet; the top of your head is facing the floor. Hold your legs straight but not tight, and keep your shoulders and neck relaxed. The weight of your head will gently stretch the muscles of your neck so it is important to be aware of the position of your head, allowing it to hang freely between your arms. If you are unable to reach the floor with your hands, do not strain or over-extend your body in an attempt to do so, as this can result in damage to your hamstrings and back. It is more important to be aware that you are relaxed, and that your body is stretching to its natural capacity.

4 The Equestrian Pose: *Ashwa Sanchalanasana*

Breathe in and take your right leg back so that the toes and the knee are on the floor. The left leg is bent and your left foot is flat on the floor. Place your hands on the floor either side of your left foot. In this posture the lunge is deep into your hip as you lean forward over your left leg, while a full extension is felt throughout your right hip and leg.

5 The Plank: *Santolanasana*

This movement is the way to progress from the Equestrian pose to the Mountain pose. If Salute to the Sun is done quickly I usually omit the Plank, as its benefits come from holding the position rather than moving through it quickly.

Exhale as you take your left leg back. Your feet can be together or slightly apart. Relax your neck and shoulders, holding the pose where you feel it the strongest. Do not lower your back from the straight position or lift your hips

upwards, as although these make it easier to hold for longer, they are not the correct position. You are better to hold it correctly for a shorter time and gain the most from this strenuous posture. The back is held straight and the heels are drawn backwards for the full stretch. For the most benefit hold this position while you breathe. This posture greatly improves strength in your wrists and arms and if you are weak in these areas regular practice will very quickly improve your strength.

6 The Mountain (or Downward Dog): *Parvatasana*

Hold the Plank for as long as you can, but never straining, then lift the hips up and drop your head down between the shoulders. Draw your hips back away from your hands, thereby obtaining a deep stretch throughout your legs, back and arms. Ease the heels towards the floor. The weight is towards the legs—feel a full extension throughout your back and legs. As greater flexibility is achieved, your heels will come closer to the floor without changing the position of your feet or your hands.

7 The Salute with Eight Limbs: *Ashtang Ganarnaskra*

As you breathe out, lower your body to the floor. Touch the floor with your toes, knees, chest, chin and hands. This position gets its name because eight parts of your body are touching the floor. The

pelvis, hips and abdominal area should not be in contact with the floor. This movement is the way to progress from position 6 to position 8.

8 The Cobra: *Bhujangasana*

Breathe in as you straighten your arms and lift your body from the floor. This will form an arch in your back. Do not arch your back further than is comfortable as this will only cause tension. If you are not very loose or flexible in the back, your arms can remain slightly bent in the final position, or you can practise the Sphinx here until your suppleness and flexibility have improved. With time and practice your back will gradually loosen so that your arms can be straightened. Your hips and pelvis remain in contact with the floor, and your head is taken back only if you have the flexibility to do so, and are free from injury or tension in your neck.

9 The Mountain: *Parvatasana*

Breathe out and return to position 6.

10 The Equestrian Pose: *Ashwa Sanchalanasana*

Breathe in and return to position 4, stepping your left foot in between your hands as your right leg is extended back. If this movement is difficult come onto your knees after the Mountain and then step the left foot through.

11 Forward Bend: *Padahastasana*

Breathe out as you step both feet together. Keep your head down with your neck, shoulders and arms relaxed. Your legs remain straight and relaxed in the forward bend, as in position 3.

12 Raised Arms: *Hasta Uttanasana*

Breathe in as your body is raised to the upright standing position, taking your arms above your head, arching back slightly to repeat position 2.

If you have a weak or injured back, I recommend bending your knees slightly as you return to the standing position when moving from position 11 to position 12, or have your feet apart a little to reduce the stretch slightly. This will help prevent extra strain on your back muscles, while it greatly reduces the extent of the stretch in your hamstrings.

Breathe out for the final posture, bringing the palms of your hands together at the centre of your chest to return to the Prayer position. Your body is straight and relaxed.

This completes half a round of Salute to the Sun. Continue on, remembering to take your left leg back in positions 4 and 10 for the second side to give equal stretch to both sides of your body.

When you have completed the number of full rounds you wish to do, always rest on the floor in a relaxation position or the Corpse, or with your knees bent if you are experiencing discomfort in the lower back, until your breathing and heart rate have returned to normal. When you feel quiet and relaxed take a few slow, deep yoga breaths and visualise prana moving through your body, mind and spirit.

The following chapter presents six suggested groupings of exercises to use in completing your postnatal exercise program. I hope you continue to enjoy your yoga practices, and find a place for yoga on life's busy path. May your life always be blessed with many special moments and wonderful adventures as you share this unique and precious journey together, as mother and child.

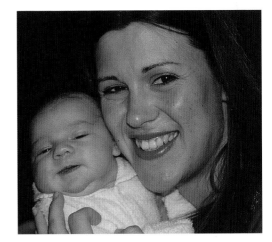

CHAPTER 24

SIX POSTNATAL EXERCISE PROGRAMS

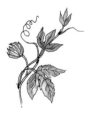

Before you begin any of these programs, which are designed to be used from six months after the birth, always spend 5 to 10 minutes in a relaxation pose of your choice, either sitting up or lying on your back. Close your eyes and bring your awareness to the natural breath. When you are ready, do some slow deep cleansing breaths followed by another breathing exercise or breath awareness exercise. On completion of the program, finish with a choice of breathing exercises, meditation or yoga nidra. Remember to do at least 100 pelvic floor exercises every day.

Program 1

1. Standing:
   Exercises for the hands (page 65)
   Shoulder rotations (page 67)
   Chest expansion exercises for the arms (page 67)
   Head and neck exercises (page 66)
2. Easy Spinal Twist (page 58)
3. Salute to the Sun (page 212). Do this three to five times slowly, or three times slowly and three times faster, in conjunction with the breathing. Rest on completion until your breathing and heart rate have returned to normal. Stretch and return to a standing position.
4. Heavenly Stretch (page 69)
5. Side bend (page 71)
6. Hero Pose (page 73)
7. Warrior Pose (page 75)
8. Wide-A Leg Stretch (page 76)
9. Rest in the Child Pose (page 63)

Program 2

1. Standing:
   Exercises for the hands (page 65)
   Shoulder rotations (page 67)
   Chest expansion exercises for the arms (page 67)
   Head and neck exercises (page 66)
2. Easy Spinal Twist (page 58)
3. Salute to the Sun (page 212). Do this three to five times slowly, or three times slowly and three times faster, in conjunction with the breathing. Rest on completion until your breathing and heart rate have returned to normal. Stretch and return to a standing position.
4. Heavenly Stretch (page 69)
5. The Tree balance (page 80), Dynamic Tree balance (page 81)
6. Eagle Balance Pose (page 82)
7. Standing squatting exercises and postures, including the Deep Standing Squat (page 51) and Chopping Wood (page 53).
8. Sitting on the floor:
   Exercises for the feet (page 25)
   Hip rotations (page 27)
   Butterfly pose (page 28)
   Sitting on the floor or a stool and do the other squatting exercises (page 47)
9. Rest in the Sleeping Tortoise (page 148)

Program 3

1. Standing:

   Exercises for the hands (page 65)

   Shoulder rotations (page 67)

   Chest expansion exercises for the arms (page 67)

   Head and neck exercises (page 66)

2. Easy Spinal Twist (page 58)

3. Salute to the Sun (page 212). Do this three to five times slowly, or three times slowly and three times faster, in conjunction with the breathing. Rest on completion until your breathing and heart rate have returned to normal. Stretch and return to a standing position.

4. Heavenly Stretch (page 69)

5. Pelvic rocking (page 37), the Cat and the Tiger (page 40). Rest in the Child pose (page 63).

6. The Head to Knee pose (page 198)

7. The seated spinal twists (page 58)

8. Hip rotations (page 27) and the Half Butterfly (page 28)

9. The seated wide leg exercises (page 31), including Churning the Mill (page 33)

10. The spinal twists resting on your back (page 61). Follow by relaxing with the knees bent and rocking from side to side.

11. With your feet against the wall practise the Plough Preparation Pose (page 200),

    followed by the Half Shoulder Stand (page 202) and the Plough (page 205). On completion bring your knees into your chest and rock from side to side.

12. The Pelvic Tilt (page 43) or the Shoulder Pose (page 210). Complete a suitable counter-pose, for example the Child Pose (page 63), Pelvic Rocking (page 37) or the Cat (page 40).

Program 4

1. Standing:

   Exercises for the hands (page 65)

   Shoulder rotations (page 67)

   Chest expansion exercises for the arms (page 67)

   Head and neck exercises (page 66)

2. Easy Spinal Twist (page 58)

3. Salute to the Sun (page 212). Do this three to five times slowly, or three times slowly and three times faster, in conjunction with the breathing. Rest on completion until your breathing and heart rate have returned to normal. Stretch and return to a standing position.

4. Heavenly Stretch pose (page 69)

5. Practice the Mountain Pose (page 78) and hold it for 10 natural breaths or longer if you wish. Rest in the Child Pose (page 63) before repeating the Mountain.

6. The Cat and the Tiger (page 40)

7. The Sphinx (page 208), the Cobra (page 215) and the Bow (page 210), resting between each one into the Child Pose.

8. Pelvic Rocking (page 37), then rest in the Child Pose

Program 5

1. Standing:

   Exercises for the hands (page 65)

   Shoulder rotations (page 67)

   Chest expansion exercises for the arms (page 67)

   Head and neck exercises (page 66)

2. Easy Spinal Twist (page 58)

3. Salute to the Sun (page 212). Do this three to five times slowly, or three times slowly and three times faster, in conjunction with the breathing. Rest on completion until your breathing and heart rate have returned to normal. Stretch and return to a standing position.

4. Heavenly Stretch (page 69)

5. Resting on your back, do the Easy Spinal Twist (page 61) and the Full Spinal Twist (page 62).

6. The abdominal exercises (page 193), including the Boat Pose (page 199) and Rowing the Boat (page 197).

7. The Head to Knee Pose (page 198), followed by the Pelvic Tilt (page 43).

8. The Dynamic Plough (page 206): repeat variation 1 ten times and rest until your breathing has returned to normal.

9. Practice variation 2 of the Dynamic Plough five times. Rest, then hold the knees into the chest and rock from side to side.

10. The Pelvic Tilt (page 43) or the Shoulder Pose (page 210)

11. Relaxation pose of your choice

Program 6

1. Standing:

   Exercises for the hands (page 65)

   Shoulder rotations (page 67)

   Chest expansion exercises for the arms (page 67)

   Head and neck exercises (page 66)

2. Easy Spinal Twist (page 58)

3. Salute to the Sun (page 212). Do this three to five times slowly, or three times slowly and three times faster, in conjunction with the breathing. Rest on completion until your breathing and heart rate have returned to normal.

Stretch and return to a standing position.

4. Heavenly Stretch pose (page 69)

5. Practise the Head of the Cow (page 40) and other arm exercises (pages 39-40).

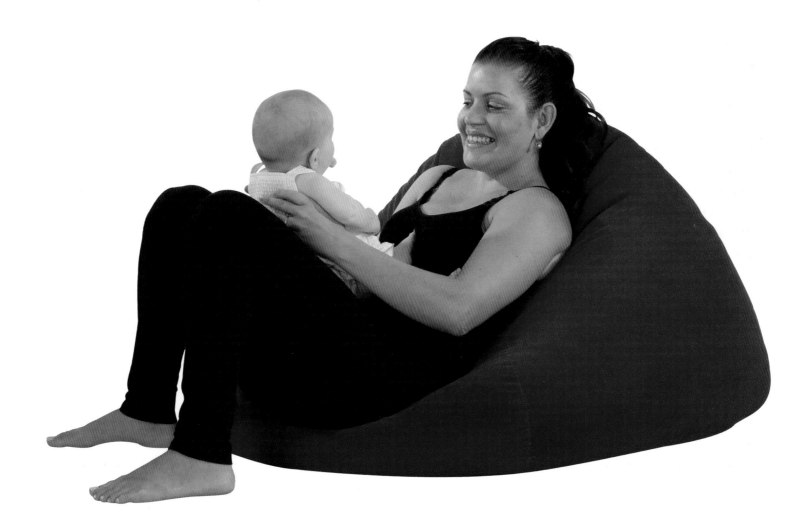

RECOMMENDED READING

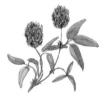

Airola, Paavo, 1979, *Every Woman's Book*, Health Plus,, Sherwood, OR

Balaskas, Janet, 1989, *New Active Birth*, Thorsons Publishing Group, London

Balaskas, Janet, 2004, *The Water Birth Book*, Thorsons Publishing Group, London

Beale, Cheryl, 1999, *Pregnancy: A guide to natural therapies*, Hill of Content, Melbourne

Bolen, Jean Shinoda, 1994, *Crossing to Avalon: A woman's midlife pilgrimage*, HarperCollins, San Francisco

Buckley, Dr Sarah, 2005, *Gentle Birth, Gentle Mothering*, One Moon Press, Brisbane.

Charmine, Susan E. (ed.) 1989, *The Complete Book of Juice Therapy*, Thorsons Publishing Group, London

Choedzong, Sakya Losal, 1996, *Samatha Meditation*, Tibetan Buddhist Society of Canberra, Canberra

Capacchione, Lucia, PhD, ATR & Sandra Bardsley RN, FACCE, 1994, *Creating a Joyful Birth Experience*, Fireside Press, New York

Chopra, Deepak, 1990, *Perfect Health*, Bantam Books, London.

Chopra, Deepak, 1993, *Creating Affluence*, New World Library, Novato, CA

Chopra, Deepak, 1994, *The Seven Spiritual Laws of Success*, Amber-Allen Publishing, San Rafael, CA

Chopra, Deepak, 2005, *Magical Beginnings, Enchanted Lives*, Random House, New York

Dalai Lama, 1992, *Selected Words of His Holiness the Dalai Lama*, Margaret Gee, Sydney

Dalai Lama, 1994, *The Way to Freedom*, HarperCollins, New York

Dyer, Wayne, 1997, *Manifest Your Destiny*, HarperCollins, New York

Emoto, Masaru, 2001, *The Message from Water*, Hado Publishing, Tokyo and Torrance, CA

Emoto, Masaru, 2006, *Love Thyself: The message from water III*, Hay House, London

England, Pam & Rob Horowitz, 1998, *Birthing From Within*, Partera Press, Independent Publishers Group, Chicago

Fontana, David, 1993, *The Secret Language of Symbols*, Pavilion Books, London

Hall, Dorothy, 1976, *The Natural Health Book*, Nelson, Melbourne

Hall, Dorothy, 1980, *The Dorothy Hall Herb Tea Book*, The Pythagorean Press, Sydney

Hamlin, Catherine, 2005, *The Hospital by the River: A story of hope*, Pan Macmillan, Sydney

Hutchinson, Ronald, 1974, *Yoga: A way of life*, Hamlyn, Middlesex

Iyengar, B.K.S., 1966, *Light on Yoga*, George Allen & Unwin, London

Jensen, Bernard, 1978, *Nature Has a Remedy*, Bernard Jensen, USA

Kenton, L. & S., 1986, *Raw Energy*, Doubleday, Sydney

Khyentse, Dilgo, 1994, *The Wish Fulfilling Jewel*, Shambhala, Boston

Sheila Kitzinger, 2003, *The New Pregnancy and Childbirth*, Dorling Kindersley, London

Kloss, Jethro, 1946, *Back to Eden*, Back to Eden Books, California

Krystal, Phyllis, 1989, *Cutting the Ties that Bind*, Element Books, Longmead, UK

Last, Walter, 1977, *Heal Yourself*, Health Print, New Zealand

Lipson, Tony, 1994, *From Conception to Birth: Our most important journey*, Millennium Books, Sydney

Naish, F. & J. Roberts, 1996, *The Natural Way to Better Babies*, Random House, Sydney

Price, Catherine & Sandra Robinson, 2005, *Birth: Conceiving, nurturing and giving birth to your baby*, Pan Macmillan, Sydney

Shri Yogendra, 1977, *Hatha Yoga Simplified*, The Yoga Institute, Bombay

Sogyal Rinpoche, 1994a, *Meditation*, Rider Books, London.

Sogyal Rinpoche, 1994b, *The Tibetan Book of Living and Dying*, Rider Books, London.

Swami Satyananda Saraswati, 1978, *Yoga Nidra, Deep Relaxation*, Satyananda Ashrams Australia, Gosford, NSW

Swami Satyananda Saraswati, 1985, *Kundalini Tantra*, Satyananda Ashrams Australia, Gosford, NSW

Vogel, H.C.A. 1990, *The Nature Doctor*, Mainstream, Edinburgh

Walker, Barbara, 1983, *The Women's Encyclopedia of Myths and Secrets*, HarperCollins, New York

Walker, Barbara, 1995, *The Women's Dictionary of Symbols and Sacred Objects*, HarperCollins, New York

Wimala, Bhante Y., 1998, *Lessons of the Lotus*, Judy Piatkus Ltd, London

INDEX

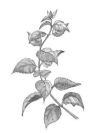